10/06

Ohmer

Respiratory Care

Dedication

For my daughter Carys who has endured much in the writing
of this book.

Respiratory Care

Caia Francis
MSc, CBiol, MIBiol, BSc (Hons), AKC,
RGN, PGCE, Asthma Diploma
Senior Lecturer
University of the West of England
Bristol

Blackwell
Publishing

© 2006 by Blackwell Publishing Ltd

Editorial offices:
Blackwell Publishing Ltd, 9600 Garsington Road, Oxford OX4 2DQ, UK
    Tel: +44 (0)1865 776868
Blackwell Publishing Inc., 350 Main Street, Malden, MA 02148-5020, USA
    Tel: +1 781 388 8250
Blackwell Publishing Asia Pty Ltd, 550 Swanston Street, Carlton, Victoria
3053, Australia
    Tel: +61 (0)3 8359 1011

First published 2006 by Blackwell Publishing Ltd

ISBN-13: 978-1-4051-1717-3
ISBN-10: 1-4051-1717-6

Library of Congress Cataloging-in-Publication Data
Francis, Caia.
    Respiratory care / Caia Francis.
      p. ; cm.
    Includes bibliographical references and index.
    ISBN-13: 978-1-4051-1717-3 (alk. paper)
    ISBN-10: 1-4051-1717-6 (alk. paper)
    1. Respiratory organs–Diseases–Patients–Medical care.
  2. Respiratory therapy.   3. Respiratory organs–Diseases–Nursing.
I Title.
    [DNLM: 1. Respiratory Tract Diseases.   2. Patient Care.   WF 140
  F818r 2006]

RC731.F73 2006
616.2′004231–dc22

                                                                 2005013041

A catalogue record for this title is available from the British Library

Set in 9 on 11 pt Palatino by SNP Best-set Typesetter Ltd., Hong Kong
Printed and bound in India by Gopsons Papers Ltd, New Delhi.

For further information on Blackwell Publishing, visit our website:
www.blackwellnursing.com

Contents

Preface

The world health organisation estimates that in 2005 respiratory illness affects at least seven million people world-wide. This figure is expected to increase as respiratory illnesses such as tuberculosis (TB) and chronic obstructive pulmonary disease (COPD) become more prevalent.

This book succinctly addresses the key issues required to deliver excellent respiratory care for today's patients. Each chapter utilises an evidenced-based approach, clearly outlining the research supporting the rationale for the principles of patient care. Where appropriate, consideration is given to both national and international guidelines that are routinely referred to when providing care for the respiratory patient.

It is essential reading for both pre and post registration health care professionals currently working with respiratory patients and those who intend to work in this area. Providing evidence for clinical practice and increased awareness of issues pertinent to both patients and their families. It is suitable for both health care professionals working within a hospital or community setting.

It will also act as a reference for the care of patients with major respiratory illnesses, and as an introductory text for those who wish to further their respiratory knowledge. Each chapter seeks to not only cover the key issues of respiratory care but to also provide enough detail to extend clinical practice and knowledge beyond a basic level.

The major respiratory illnesses are considered in detail: including COPD; asthma; lung cancer and TB. Other chapters include a comprehensive consideration of the use of oxygen therapy, respiratory patient assessment and the use of nebulisers and inhalers.

Each chapter is clearly written, with bullet points emphasising fundamental issues. Summaries at the end of each chapter provide both quick reference for the chapter and as a guide for revision of the topic. Case studies are used throughout as examples of both good and poor respiratory patient care, aiding understanding of the chapter and providing points for discussion and consideration.

A patient centred focus is used to help health care professionals develop a greater understanding of the problems those with respiratory illnesses endure. Thus aiding health care professionals to take an empathetic approach in their daily interactions with both patients and their families.

The book is expected to become essential reading for all whom wish to develop or extend their knowledge of respiratory patient care. Providing a firm, evidenced based basis for excellent patient centred clinical practice.

Acknowledgements

I would like to thank my parents for their limitless help in proof reading, specifically my father for his dedication, and my husband for his continual support, especially with Chapter 6. And all the people that I have cared for and worked with who have helped shap my interest in respiratory nursing, in particular, Dr Huw Thomas.

Anatomy and Physiology of the Respiratory System | **1**

The primary function of the respiratory system is to facilitate the entry of oxygen into the bloodstream and allow the coincidental loss of carbon dioxide from that system. The respiratory system has to have the ability to respond quickly to demands of the body and plays a critical role in the restoration and preservation of homeostasis in the tissues. The anatomy and morphology of the respiratory system has not only evolved to support its primary function, but in addition has also evolved to support other functions that are vital in maintaining the body's integrity. Such important and crucial roles include: aiding in the maintenance of the body's acid–base balance; metabolism of specific compounds; filtering unwanted materials from the circulation; prevention and reduction of infection and acting as a reservoir for blood (West 2000).

The main aim of this chapter is to examine the premise that the major purpose of the respiratory system is to provide the opportunity for inspired air to come into close proximity with the circulating blood thus allowing diffusion to occur (Bourke 2003). The rate of that diffusion will be in accord with Fick's law of diffusion (see Table 1.1).

It can be seen that Fick's law defines the essential morphology and physiology of the lung. Thus it is predictable that the region of the respiratory system which allows gas exchange to occur will have a thin sheet of tissue between the inspired air and the circulating blood. These regions within the lungs are known as alveoli.

This chapter aims to:

❏ Provide an overview of the gross anatomy of the respiratory system.
❏ Review the key physiological principles of the respiratory system and related aspects of the cardiovascular system including: ventilation; perfusion; mechanics of breathing; the control of breathing; the transport of gases within the cardiovascular system.

STRUCTURE OF THE RESPIRATORY SYSTEM

The major components of the respiratory system are two lungs set within the thoracic cage. The right lung is divided into three lobes, upper middle and lower, and the left lung into two lobes.

Table 1.1 Fick's law of diffusion.

Solutes and ions move randomly in all directions and the consequence is that in a non-homogeneous solution such random movement will result in a net movement of solute from regions of high concentration towards regions of lower concentration, i.e. the effective net movement is down a concentration gradient.

Molecules of a gas also move randomly and will thus tend to distribute themselves equally in an enclosed space. The net movement of molecules will be from regions of high partial pressure towards regions with a lower partial pressure, i.e. net movement is dependent on a partial pressure difference. The rate of diffusion of a specific gas through any gas is very much greater than the rate of diffusion through a liquid. It is often quoted that the rate of diffusion of CO_2 through air is 10 000 times greater than its diffusion rate through water. Even so because of the constant collisions between gas molecules they do not move directly, taking minutes or hours to move across an average room.

The rates of diffusion of gasses through a 'porous body' are inversely proportional to the square root of their molecular weights (Graham's law).

Thus molecules of hydrogen (H_2) will diffuse at $4\times$ the rate of oxygen molecules (O_2).

Fick's first law of diffusion states that the amount of gas (J_{net}) that moves across a sheet of tissue is proportional to the partial pressure gradient of the gas (C) and the area of the sheet (A) but inversely proportional to its thickness (Δx).

$J_{net} = -D.A.\Delta C/\Delta x$

Where D is the diffusion coefficient ($m^2 sec^{-1}$)

Vessels, nerves and lymphatics enter the lungs on their medial surfaces at a point known as the hilum (Cotes 1993). Each lobe is divided into a number of wedge-shaped bronchopulmonary segments with their apices at the hilum and their bases at the lung surface. Each bronchopulmonary segment can be removed surgically with little bleeding or air leakage from the remaining lung (Selby 2002).

Each lung is lined by a thin membrane, the visceral pleura that is continuous with the parietal pleura lining the chest wall, diaphragm, pericardium and mediasturnum. The space between the parietal and visceral layers is very thin in health and lubricated with pleural fluid (Ward *et al.* 2002).

Figure 1.1 illustrates the gross anatomical features of the respiratory system. The upper respiratory tract comprises the nose, pharynx and larynx. The lower respiratory tract commences with the trachea and comprises the remaining sections of respiratory tract (Ward *et al.* 2002).

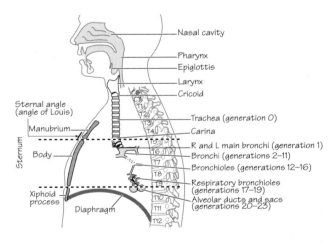

Fig. 1.1 Gross anatomical features of respiratory system. With permission from Blackwell Publishing (Ward *et al* 2002).

In fit healthy and well adults inspired air enters the respiratory tract usually via the nostrils. The mouth is an alternative route of entry but it is not usually the principal entrance for inspired air. During its passage through the respiratory airways the air is warmed and saturated with water vapour (Ganong 1993).

The inhaled air is first filtered by the nose and then any large sized inhaled particulate that remain are removed from the inspired air and deposited on the mucus coated walls of the respiratory airways. The walls of the respiratory tract are composed of ciliated columnar epithelium, mucus glands and goblet cells. The mucus glands and goblet cells secrete mucus and the cilia beat together sending waves of contraction passing in an organised manner from cell to cell. Any particles trapped in the sticky mucus layer are moved upwards and out of the lungs. This is known as the mucociliary escalator, and is an important component in the respiratory system's defence against infection (Cotes 1993). The beating of the cilia can be inhibited by the inhalation of toxins, for example tobacco smoke. The alveoli have no ciliated cells and any particles that reach this region of the lung will be removed by macrophages (cells of the immune system) and exported out of the lungs via the lymphatic system or the blood flow (Margereson 2002).

The first airway that the inspired air enters is known as the trachea. This divides into two at the level of the fifth cervical vertebrae to form the right and left bronchus (see Fig. 1.2) The right and left bronchus further subdivide into small and even smaller airways, known as bronchi and then bronchioles. Bronchi are airways with cartilage in their walls, and there are about ten divisions of such airways. The smaller airways without cartilage in their walls are the bronchioles (Ward *et al.* 2002). Bronchi make up the conducting airways of the respiratory system. No gas exchange takes place in these regions and thus they are often referred to as the anatomical dead space. The volume of air in this region is *circa* 150 mL (West 2000).

The bronchioles further lead into alveolar ducts which are completely lined with alveoli. This is the region of the lung where 'gas exchange' can occur and is known as the respiratory zone.

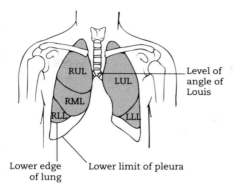

Fig. 1.2 Surface anatomy of the lungs. Anterior view. LLL, left lower lobe; LUL, left upper lobe; RLL, right lower lobe; RML, right middle lobe; RUL, right upper lobe. With permission from Blackwell Publishing (Bourke 2003).

Name	Zone number	
Trachea	0	⎫
Bronchi	2	⎬ Conducting zone =
Bronchioles	4	anatomical dead space
Terminal Bronchioles	5–16	⎭
Respiratory Bronchioles	17	⎫
Alveolar ducts	20	⎬ Transitional and
Alveolar sacs	23	⎭ respiratory zones

Fig. 1.3 Generation of the respiratory system.

Figure 1.3 illustrates the generation of the respiratory tract and outlines the conducting airways and the airways involved directly in gas exchange.

Alveoli are between 0.1 and 0.2 mm in diameter and are lined by a thin layer of cells. Two types of cells exist: type I pneumocytes and type II pneumocytes. The latter produce surfactant which is essential in reducing the surface tension of the alveoli and helps in maintaining their stability. The reduction or absence of surfactant can lead to the large forces that develop within the alveoli causing their collapse and thus their removal from gas exchange (Fig. 1.4).

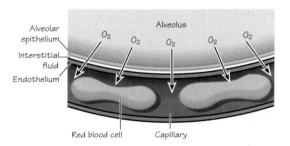

Fig. 1.4 Alveoli structure. With permission from Blackwell Publishing (Ward *et al* 2002).

MECHANICS OF BREATHING

During inspiration the volume of the thoracic cavity increases and air is drawn into the lung. The increase in volume is brought about partly by contraction of the diaphragm, which causes it to descend, and partly by the action of the intercostal muscles which raise the ribs thus increasing the cross-sectional area of the thorax (see Fig. 1.5). Inspired air flows down to about the terminal bronchioles by bulk flow. Beyond that point the combined cross sectional area of the airways is vast, such that the forward velocity of the gas becomes small. Diffusion of the gas within the airways then takes over as the dominant mechanism of ventilation within the respiratory zone.

The lung is elastic and during resting breathing, expiration occurs as it returns passively to its pre-inspiratory volume (West 2000).

Vigorous exercise, dyspnoea and other factors can result in the accessory muscles associated with breathing becoming recruited into use. These include the abdominal, sternocleido-mastoid and pectoral muscles.

CONTROL OF BREATHING

Two distinct neural mechanisms regulate respiration (Bouhuys 1977). One is responsible for voluntary control, the other for

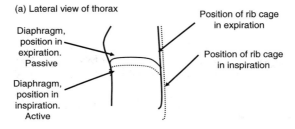

(a) Lateral view of thorax

Diaphragm, position in expiration. Passive

Position of rib cage in expiration

Position of rib cage in inspiration

Diaphragm, position in inspiration. Active

(b) Cross sectional schematic diagram of thoracic cavity, illustrating position of diaphragm in inspiration and expiration

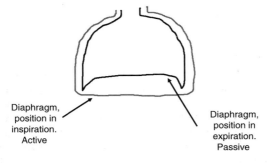

Diaphragm, position in inspiration. Active

Diaphragm, position in expiration. Passive

Fig. 1.5 Mechanics of breathing.

automatic control. The voluntary control system is located within the cerebral cortex, whereas the automatic system is located within the pons and medulla. The motor neurons to the expiratory muscles are inhibited when those supplying the inspiratory muscles are active and vice versa (Ganong 1993).

The automatic system generates a rhythmic discharge of neurons within the brain, producing the stimuli which control automatic respiration. Expiration during quiet breathing is passive, thus any control of expiration from the automatic neural system only becomes significant during fast laboured breathing.

REGULATION OF THE RESPIRATORY CENTRE

In fit healthy humans the normal stimulus to breathe is associated with a rising level of CO_2 within the blood. The concentration of CO_2 within the blood is detected within the body by central chemoreceptors, whose exact location within the brain is not known. These central chemoreceptors are stimulated when there is a rise in CO_2 that has diffused across the cerebral spinal fluid. The increase in the molar concentration of CO_2 changes the equilibria and results in a consequential increase in the concentrations of bicarbonate ions and hydrogen ions (i.e. a pH shift).

$$CO_2 + H_2O \leftrightarrow H_2CO_3 \leftrightarrow HCO_3^- + H^+$$

The hydrogen ions stimulate the neuronal control of the respiratory centre and the resulting impulses cause the muscles involved in the respiratory processes to contract thereby increasing the respiration rate (Levitzky 1999).

The second stimulus to breathe is a decrease in PO_2, i.e. a fall in oxygen concentration within the blood. This is detected by the carotid bodies (located near the carotid bifurcation) and the aortic bodies (located near the aortic arch). This stimulus often becomes the main driving mechanism in type II respiratory failure. This is sometimes referred to as the 'hypoxic drive' to breathe. Figure 1.6 summarises the main control mechanisms of respiration (West 2000, Ward *et al.* 2002).

Of course other factors can influence respiration: these include painful stimuli, inflation receptors in the lungs, triggers for sneezing, coughing, exercise, etc.

Table 1.2 illustrates the key events that occur during normal quiet inspiration and expiration.

THE WORK OF BREATHING

Energy expenditure during quiet breathing is normally less than 5% of the total body oxygen uptake, although this may increase up to 30% or more during vigorous exercise or respiratory distress (Levitzky *et al.* 1990).

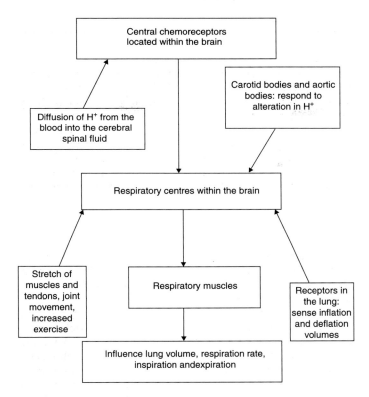

Fig. 1.6 Main control mechanisms of respiration.

Table 1.2 Key events in normal breathing.

Inspiration	Expiration
Increase CO_2 conc. within blood	Neuronal stimulation by automatic centre ceases
Stimulation of respiratory centre	Inspiratory muscles relax
Stimulation of diaphragm	Thoracic volume decreases
Increase in thoracic volume	Elastic recoil of lungs
Alveoli pressure decreases	Alveolar pressure increases
Air enters via bulk flow	Air flows out of lungs

MAINTENANCE OF AIRWAY TONE

Hormones, peptides and neurotransmitters can affect the smooth muscle lining the respiratory airway. There is a complex interplay between these factors, which minute to minute result in variations in the respiratory airway size.

The autonomic nervous system is perhaps the key player in regulating the contraction and relaxation of airway smooth muscle. Parasympathetic nerves release acetylcholine which acts upon muscarinic receptors within the smooth muscle, causing smooth muscle contraction and an increase secretion of mucus. Drugs which mimic these effects are sometimes given in bronchial challenges, e.g. metacholine. However drugs that inhibit these effects are frequently given in respiratory medicine and these include atropine and ipratropium bromide (Margareson 2002).

Sympathetic nerves release noradrenaline and their effects are also mediated by adrenaline. Smooth airway muscles have β_2 receptors which respond to adrenaline by causing relaxation of the smooth muscle. However their activation may not be as a direct response of stimulation from the sympathetic system. Recent research suggests that sympathetic nerves do not play a primary regulatory role in the relaxation of smooth muscle (Barnes 1986, 1993, 1998). Rather the circulating blood levels of adrenaline and noradrenaline are more important in causing airway smooth muscle relaxation.

Drugs that stimulate the β_2 receptors, thus initiating smooth muscle relaxation, are called β_2 agonists and include salbutamol and terbutaline.

PULMONARY CIRCULATION

The pulmonary vascular system is described as a high-volume low-pressure system (Brewis & White 1995). Resistance within the pulmonary vascular system is mainly within the arterioles and capillaries, and these can alter their dilation rapidly. Thus in the regions of the lung that become poorly oxygenated, the capillaries supplying them will constrict and divert blood to those areas that have a greater supply of oxygen. Detailed anatomy of the pulmonary circulation is outside the scope of this chapter. More information can be found in any good standard textbook of anatomy.

Pulmonary arterioles may also constrict in response to localised hypoxia. In chronic lung disease this may result in long term vasoconstriction, increased cardiac output resulting in right ventricular failure (cor pulmonale) and in many cases death (Ferguson & Cherniack 1993).

COMPOSITION OF INSPIRED AIR

Inspired atmospheric air at sea level is comprised of a number of gases. Of particular importance in respiration are:

- Nitrogen (N_2) 76%.
- Oxygen (O_2) 20.98%.
- Carbon dioxide (CO_2) 0.04%.

The balance is made up by the inert gases.

The partial pressure of water vapour is variable, usually in the range 0.2 to 2.0 kPa.

Each gas exerts a pressure (partial pressure). The sum or total of all the partial pressures of gases and partial pressure of the water vapour within the atmosphere exert a pressure known as atmospheric pressure, or barometric pressure (Dalton's law). At sea level the 'standard' atmospheric pressure is usually defined as 101 kPa.

Thus the partial pressure of nitrogen is:

$$\frac{76}{100} \times 101 \, \text{kPa} = 76.76 \, \text{kPa}$$

Oxygen's partial pressure is:

$$\frac{20.98}{100} \times 101 \, \text{kPa} = 21.19 \, \text{kPa}$$

With increasing altitude the partial pressure that each gas exerts decreases and the total atmospheric pressure falls. Roughly every rise in altitude of 550 m will halve the atmospheric pressure. Consequently those people who undertake climbing Everest (circa 8850 m) will experience a significant decrease in atmospheric pressure and an associated decrease in the partial pressure of inspired oxygen. This reduction in the amount of oxygen inspired combined with the effect of the smaller diffusion pressure gradient existing within the lungs will contribute to the risk of developing altitude sickness.

Those who engage in aeroplane travel might consider the advantages they enjoyed by being in a pressured cabin while flying at 10 000–12 000 m. Aeroplane cabins are usually pressurised to remain at the equivalent of the atmospheric pressure found at 2000–3000 m irrespective of the actual altitude of the flight. This 'simulated altitude' would usually have little effect upon the respiratory system of a fit and healthy adult; however those with abnormal or immature respiratory systems can be affected by aeroplane flight as can those who require oxygen therapy at home. Consequently guidelines have been written to aid in decisions concerning the fitness for flight and the possible consequences of aeroplane travel (British Thoracic Society (BTS) 2002).

By the time the inspired air reaches the alveoli it is fully saturated with water vapour: saturated water vapour at sea level would have a partial pressure of about 6 kPa. Thus to calculate the partial pressure of oxygen within the alveoli the partial pressure of water vapour must first be subtracted from the atmospheric pressure. Thus the pressure of oxygen within the alveoli of fit healthy individuals is usually estimated to be circa 13 kPa (Ganong 1993).

TRANSPORT OF GASES

It has been shown above that the partial pressure of oxygen within the alveoli is circa 13 kPa, while the blood returning from the right side of the heart in the pulmonary artery has a pO_2 of circa 5.7 kPa. Thus the pressure difference for oxygen within the respiratory system is such that diffusion (movement of molecules from regions of high concentration to a region of low concentration) will ensure oxygen moves from the alveoli into the blood. Conversely the concentration of CO_2 within the inspired air is lower than in the blood so that diffusion will ensure CO_2 moves from the blood into the alveoli and is then expired.

In fit healthy individuals this is usually achieved within 0.25 seconds (Riley & Cournard 1949, Sykes *et al.* 1976). Factors that influence this diffusion process are:

- Thickness of membrane which separates the gases.
- Surface area of membrane (alveoli).
- Solubility of gases.
- Partial pressure gradient of gases.
- Ventilation of alveoli.
- Perfusion of the alveoli capillaries.

Lung diseases can influence many of the above factors, for example: mucus plugging associated with asthma will reduce the ventilation of alveoli; the effective surface area of alveoli decreases in emphysema. Other co-morbidities can also influence the diffusion time and process (West 2000).

Oxygen, once it has diffused across the alveolar capillary membrane, is carried within the blood by two methods. Some 3% of the oxygen is dissolved in the plasma; the remaining 97% is bound to haemoglobin in the red blood cells to form oxy-haemoglobin. Oxygen readily combines with haemoglobin and this reaction is fully reversible. Four molecules of oxygen can combine with one haemoglobin molecule.

The percentage of haemoglobin combined with oxygen is dependent upon the concentration of oxygen available, i.e. the partial pressure of oxygen. In the regions of the body with a high partial pressure of oxygen most of the haemoglobin will be bound with oxygen. However in regions of the body with low partial pressure of oxygen, oxygen will dissociate from the haemoglobin following the laws of diffusion (Baumann *et al.* 1987). In cases of anaemia all the available haemoglobin may be bound with oxygen within the lungs but the total oxygen carrying capacity of the blood will be insufficient to meet the body's demands. This demonstrates the principle that concentration of haemoglobin within the body significantly influences the oxygen carrying capacity of the blood. Each 1 g of fully saturated haemoglobin molecule can 'hold' 1.39 cm^3 of oxygen. Thus if the haemoglobin concentration of blood is 15 g/dL then it can be estimated that the total oxygen carrying capacity for each $100\,cm^3$ of blood is $15 \times 1.39 = 20\,cm^3$ plus the oxygen dissolved within the plasma (Hsia 1998).

Factors which influence the oxygen concentration within the blood are manifold. However the commonest are: anaemia; the partial pressure of the oxygen in the alveoli; the rate of ventilation; the rate of perfusion of the alveoli; the presence of other gases (e.g. carbon monoxide which will bind to haemoglobin in favour of oxygen); temperature; and pH.

OXYHAEMOGLOBIN DISSOCIATION CURVE

The oxyhaemoglobin dissociation curve is a sigmoid (S-shaped) curve (see Fig. 1.7). If oxygen partial pressure remains above 10 kPa and below 13 kPa the saturation of haemoglobin with oxygen remains high. However once the oxygen partial pressure falls below circa 8 kPa, the saturation of haemoglobin with oxygen rapidly falls. This has a catastrophic influence upon the normal functioning of the body.

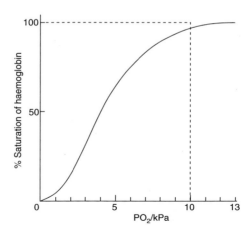

Fig. 1.7 Oxyhaemoglobin dissociation curve.

The oxyhaemoglobin dissociation curve can be influenced by a number of factors (see above). However the commonest factors which influence how haemoglobin binds with oxygen are temperature, pH and CO_2 concentration. These factors cause the curve to shift either to the left or the right (see Fig. 1.8). As can be noted by observation of this figure, a shift to the left of the oxyhaemoglobin curve will result in the haemoglobin remaining fully bound with oxygen at lower partial pressures of oxygen. Thus release of oxygen to the peripheral tissues is perhaps greater than normal; the uptake of oxygen by haemoglobin within the alveoli is reduced. A shift to the right results in oxygen unbinding from the haemoglobin at higher than usual

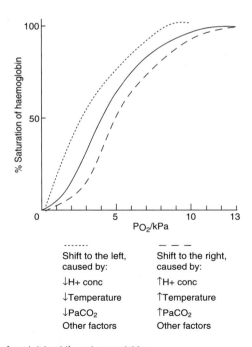

....	$-$ $-$ $-$
Shift to the left, caused by:	Shift to the right, caused by:
↓H+ conc	↑H+ conc
↓Temperature	↑Temperature
↓$PaCO_2$	↑$PaCO_2$
Other factors	Other factors

Fig. 1.8 Left and right shift oxyhaemoglobin.

partial pressure of oxygen, thus altering the amount of oxygen delivered to the peripheral tissues.

CARRIAGE OF CARBON DIOXIDE

Carbon dioxide is much more soluble in water or blood than oxygen. However although a significant amount of dissolved carbon dioxide exists in the plasma even at low pCO_2, most of the carbon dioxide transported is in the form of bicarbonate ions. Only small concentrations of the intermediate carbonic acid exist since it can rapidly dissociate to form bicarbonate and hydrogen ions (Klocke 1987).

$$CO_2 + H_2O \leftrightarrow H_2CO_3 \leftrightarrow HCO_3^- + H^+$$

Some 70% of the carbon dioxide entering the venous system is transported in the plasma, and the remaining 30% enters the red blood cells.

The carriage of carbon dioxide within the red blood cells is important. The enzyme carbonic anhydrase found within the red blood cells will considerably speed up the reaction converting the carbon dioxide and water molecules into carbonic acid molecules. As in the plasma this carbonic acid then speedily dissociates to form the bicarbonate and hydrogen ions. The overall reaction is quicker than the identical reactions that occur within the plasma.

In the red blood cells some of the carbon dioxide will also combine with amino groups of the proteins to form carbamino-CO_2. The concentration of hydrogen ions and bicarbonate ions will continue to increase in red blood cells as more carbon dioxide is unloaded from the metabolically active tissues into the veins. While bicarbonate anions will diffuse from the erythrocytes into the blood plasma the erythrocyte cell membrane is relatively impermeable to H^+ and other cations such as Na^+ or K^+. Some of the hydrogen ions will complex with the haemoglobin while chloride ions diffuse from the plasma in exchange for the bicarbonate ions and in effect balance the charges on remaining hydrogen cations. The number of osmotically active ions in the erythrocytes has thus increased as a result of the chain of reactions that followed the uptake of CO_2 into the cells. Water molecules will now move into the cell, the consequential effects being the dilution of the molecular and ionic concentrations and a small increase in the volume of the erythrocytes.

It is generally regarded that the 'total CO_2 content of the blood' may be quantified as being equivalent to the sum of the dissolved carbon dioxide, plus the carbon dioxide that could be released from the bicarbonate and carbonate anions together with that transported as the carbamino-CO_2.

All the above reactions are fully reversible and in the lung they form a system which ensures that carbon dioxide is released from the arterial blood after entering the lung via the Pulmonary artery. The carbon dioxide released then moves by diffusion from the blood into the alveoli of the lungs.

Respiratory acidosis is said to occur when the total dissolved CO_2 is higher than its normal limits. Respiratory alkalosis is said to occur when the total dissolved CO_2 is too low. (Note the effect of CO_2 concentration on the equilibrium reached in the reactions given above, particularly with reference to the changes that would occur in H^+ concentration.)

ACID–BASE BALANCE

The body is continuously producing acids as a consequence of:

- the catabolism of carbohydrates, proteins and nucleic acids;
- the conversion of metabolically produced CO_2 to carbonic acid;
- the release of lactic and other acids formed during anaerobic catabolism (West 2000).

These organic acids will partially dissociate to increase the H^+ concentration of the blood.

The general metabolic activity of the body can adjust to maintain homeostasis and compensate for any further tendency to increase the concentration of hydrogen ions by utilising its capacity to produce hydrogen ion acceptors. In general those compounds within the body that act as hydrogen ion (H^+) acceptors will either tend to increase in concentration when the pH falls or decrease in concentration as the pH rises.

There are three major systems that exist to deal with this fluctuating situation:

1. The buffer base: for example bicarbonate, proteins and phosphates are compounds that are able to accept hydrogen ions to form weak acids. This mechanism is activated almost immediately.
2. The respiratory system: the lungs will either remove or retain CO_2 depending upon the 'need' to increase or decrease CO_2 concentration. This mechanism follows the changes in the buffer system fairly quickly. Thus a fall in blood pH (i.e. a rise in H^+) will drive the equilibria towards the left to increase the pCO_2. This increase in pCO_2 will in turn increase the respiration rate and thus remove more CO_2 from the blood until a new equilibrium is established. Hyperventilation and hypoventilation have rapid effects on concentration of carbon dioxide in the blood.
3. The renal system: the renal tubules are able to retain bicarbonate or hydrogen ions or secrete them. This system response is the slowest but it is the most efficient.

The respiratory systems have other important functions, such as defence against infection, metabolism of active compounds from the body, etc. Further information concerning these functions can be found in detailed texts on the physiology and immunology of the respiratory system.

SUMMARY

❏ The respiratory system's main function is to facilitate gas exchange thus ensuring that adequate oxygen and carbon dioxide tensions are maintained within the body.
❏ Other functions of the respiratory system include allowing speech to occur; defence against infection; blood storage; acid–base balance.
❏ The structure of the respiratory system in fit healthy individuals ensures that adequate gas exchange occurs.
❏ In quiet breathing inspiration is active, involving the use of the diaphragm to increase the thoracic volume, and expiration is passive.

❑ In dyspnoea, laboured breathing or during exercise, both inspiration and expiration are active energy dependent components of respiration.

❑ Control of breathing is via two mechanisms: one automatic, the other under voluntary control.

❑ The automatic control of breathing is based upon neural impulses that are generated rhythmically within the brain.

❑ Factors that influence the control of breathing via the autonomic system are the concentration of hydrogen ions and the partial pressure of oxygen.

❑ Carriage of carbon dioxide within the body occurs within the plasma, and red blood cells.

❑ Carriage of oxygen around the body is primarily affected by the oxygen being bound to haemoglobin within the red blood cells.

❑ The oxygen dissociation curve graphically represents unloading of oxyhaemoglobin in those regions of the body with a low partial pressure of oxygen.

❑ Factors that influence the unloading and loading of oxygen with haemoglobin are temperature, pH, and atmospheric pressure.

REFERENCES

Barnes PJ (1986) Neural control of human airways in health and disease. *American Review of Respiratory Disease* **134**: 1289–1314.

Barnes PJ (1993) Non adrenergic non cholinergic nerves in airways. In: Andrews P, Widdicombe J (eds) *Pathophysiology of the gut and airways. An introduction*. Portland Press, London.

Barnes PJ (1998) Pharmacology of airway smooth muscle. *American Journal of Respiratory and Critical Care Medicine* **158** (5) 3: S123–132.

Baumann R, Bartels H, Bauer C (1987) Blood oxygen transport. In: Farhi LE, Tenney SM (eds) Gas exchange. Handbook of physiology, Section 3: The respiratory system. *American Physiological Society* **4**: 147–172.

Bouhys A (1977) *The physiology of breathing*. Grune & Stratton, New York.

Bourke SJ (2003) *Respiratory medicine*. Blackwell Publishing, Oxford.

Brewis RAL, White FE (1995) Anatomy of the thorax. In: Brewis RAL, Corrin B, Geddes DM, Gibson GJ (eds) *Respiratory medicine*. WB Saunders, London.

British Thoracic Society (2002) Managing passengers with respiratory disease planning air travel: BTS recommendations. *Thorax* **57**: 289–304.

Cotes JE (1993) *Lung function*, 5th edn. Blackwell Science, Oxford.

Ferguson GT, and Cherniack RM (1993) Management of chronic obstructive pulmonary disease. *New England Journal of Medicine* **328**: 1017–1022.

Ganong WF (1993) *Review of medical physiology*. McGraw Hill, New York.

Hsia CCW (1998) Respiratory function of hemoglobin. *New England Journal of Medicine* **338**: 239–247.

Levitzky MG (1999) *Pulmonary physiology*, 5th edn. McGraw Hill, New York.

Levitzky MG, Cairo JM, Hall SM (1990) *Introduction to respiratory care*. WB Saunders, London.

Margereson C (2002) Anatomy and physiology. In: Esmond G (ed.) *Respiratory nursing*. Bailliere Tindall, Edinburgh.

Riley RL, Cournand A (1949) Ideal alveolar air and the analysis of ventilation – perfusion relationships in the lung. *Journal of Applied Physiology* **1**: 825–847.

Schwartz AR, Smith PL, Kashima HK, Proctor DF (1994) Respiratory function of the upper airways. In: Murry JF, Nadel JA (eds) *Textbook of respiratory medicine*. Saunders, Philadelphia.

Selby C (2002) *Respiratory medicine*. Churchill Livingstone, Edinburgh.

Sykes MK, McNicol NW, Campbell EJM (1976) *Respiratory failure*, 2nd edn. Blackwell Science, Oxford.

Ward JPT, Ward J, Weiner CM, Leach RM (2002) *The respiratory system at a glance*. Blackwell Publishing, Oxford.

West JB (1995) *Pulmonary pathophysiology: the essentials*, 5th edn. Lippincott Williams & Wilkins, Philadelphia.

West JB (2000) *Respiratory physiology essentials*, 6th edn. Lippincott Williams & Wilkins, Philadelphia.

Widdicombe J, Davies A (1991) *Respiratory physiology*, 2nd edn. Edward Arnold, London.

Asthma

2

The incidence, prevalence and severity of asthma are all increasing, with childhood asthma becoming even more common (Anderson *et al.* 1994, Ryan & Freeman 2001, ISAAC 1998). There are varying estimates as to the rate of this increase in incidence, but over fifteen years the annual numbers of recorded new cases may have increased by as much as 70% (Lewis *et al.* 1996). At present it is cited as the most common chronic disease in childhood, with an estimated prevalence of between 8 and 14% (Ryan & Freeman 2001).

Within the age range 12–14 years of age, the United Kingdom has the highest incidence of asthma in the world (ISAAC 1998). World-wide the morbidity and mortality of asthma is increasing with such vigour that the management of asthma is under constant scrutiny (Chee *et al.* 1996). This crisis drives the primary health carers' demand for the publication and implementation of guidelines on asthma management (BTS SIGN 2003).

This chapter aims to:
❏ Provide a definition of asthma.
❏ Describe the effects that asthma has upon the respiratory system.
❏ Identify the common symptoms experienced by those with asthma.
❏ Identify the prevalence and incidence of asthma morbidity and mortality within the UK.
❏ Outline how asthma is managed or treated in both primary and secondary care.
❏ Consider the BTS SIGN (2003) asthma management guidelines.

Table 2.1 Definitions of asthma.

'Asthma is a chronic inflammatory disorder of the airway in which many cells play a role, in particular mast cells, eosinophils, and T-lymphocytes. In susceptible individuals this inflammation causes recurrent episodes of wheezing, breathlessness, chest tightness, and cough particularly at night and/or in the early morning. These symptoms are usually associated with widespread but variable airflow limitation that is at least partly reversible either spontaneously or with treatment. The inflammation also causes an associated increase in airway responsiveness to a variety of stimuli.' (International Consensus report on the diagnosis and management of asthma 1992)

'Asthma is a common and chronic inflammatory condition of the airways whose cause is not completely understood. As a result of inflammation the airways are hyper-responsive and they narrow easily in response to a wide range of stimuli. This may result in coughing, wheezing, chest tightness, and shortness of breath and these symptoms are often worse at night. Narrowing of the airways is usually reversible, but in some patients with chronic asthma the inflammation may lead to irreversible airflow obstruction. Characteristic pathological features include: the presence in the airway of inflammatory cells; plasma exudates; oedema; smooth muscle hypertrophy; mucus plugging, and shedding of the epithelium.' (BTS 1997.)

'Asthma is a chronic inflammatory disorder of the airways. In susceptible individuals this inflammation causes recurrent episodes of coughing, wheezing, chest tightness and difficult breathing. Inflammation makes the airways sensitive to stimuli such as allergens, chemical irritants, tobacco smoke, cold air or exercise. When exposed to these stimuli, the airways may become swollen, constricted, filled with mucus and hyper-responsive to a variety of stimuli. The resulting airflow limitation is reversible (but not completely so in some patients), either spontaneously or with treatment. When asthma therapy is adequate, inflammation can be reduced over the long term, symptoms can be controlled and most asthma related problems prevented.' (GINA 1995)

❏ Consider the current medication of asthma and future asthma therapy developments.

DEFINITION OF ASTHMA

Asthma has been defined in the past by criteria based upon its symptoms, such as the presence of wheezing signifying the existence of (variable) airflow obstruction. However current definitions consider asthma to be more than the presence of wheezing and they attempt to encapsulate the underlying pathology associated with asthma. Table 2.1 provides a resume of the current definitions of asthma.

These definitions have a high degree of commonality: they all agree that the symptoms of asthma are variable and usually reversible; can be self-limiting although usually require treatment; involve respiratory airways becoming more sensitive to stimuli resulting in airway inflammation and associated airflow obstruction.

The exact causes of asthma are not fully known at present. However in the last thirty years more is understood concerning the inflammation that occurs in asthmatic airways. This has revealed some of the possible mechanisms that may result in the physiological changes that provoke an asthma attack in susceptible individuals. Risk factors that are significant in the possible development of asthma are manifold. They include a family history of: allergy; asthma; hay fever; or eczema. In these cases it is likely that the individual with asthma is atopic (has an immune system highly responsive to allergens). (See Chapter 3, Table 3.4, which outlines the differential diagnosis of asthma and COPD.) Other risk factors include: allergen exposure; frequent respiratory tract infections, such as those caused by respiratory syncytial virus (RSV); smoking and chronic stress.

The acute and chronic inflammatory process of asthma is characterised by infiltration of the airway wall by a myriad of cells of the immune system. In the acute phase there are increases in: T-lymphocytes, eosinophils, monocytes/macrophages and mast cells. The chronic phase of asthma is associated with plasma extravasation and oedema, infiltration of the airway wall epithelium and desquamation of the airway wall epithelium. This process is controlled by cytokines (extracellular signalling proteins derived from activated white blood cells), by IgE (immunoglobulin E) and other factors. If these 'components' are measured in asthmatic patients experiencing an asthma attack, they are usually found to be present in higher concentrations than in non-asthmatic individuals. Figure 2.1 illustrates the airway remodelling that occurs in those patients with asthma.

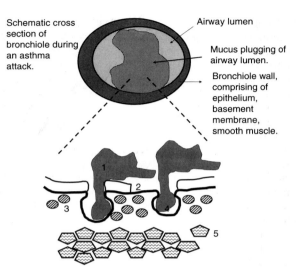

Schematic cross section of bronchiole during an asthma attack.

Airway lumen

Mucus plugging of airway lumen.

Bronchiole wall, comprising of epithelium, basement membrane, smooth muscle.

Figure 2.1 Airway remodelling in asthma patient. 1. Increased mucus production; 2. Epithelial cell desquamation and disruption (epithelial cells breaking off/missing from airway lumen); 3. Increased number of fibroblasts; 4. Goblet cell hyperplasia (increase in size and number); 5. Increased airway smooth muscle thickness. These inflammatory effects result in airways becoming more sensitive to stimuli such as pollen, animal dander, exercise and obstruction due to mucus plugging and/or smooth muscle contraction in an acute asthma attack.

Asthma thus causes profound changes to the respiratory airways, and these changes are believed to be responsible for the clinical signs and symptoms that indicate an individual may have asthma. These effects are spread throughout the whole respiratory system and are not limited to the airways involved directly in gas exchange (see Chapter 1).

DIAGNOSIS OF ASTHMA
Clinically the diagnosis of asthma is based upon the patient's medical history, physical examination and respiratory function

tests. Clinical features of asthma are recurrent episodes of wheezing, chest tightness, cough and shortness of breath. However, asthmatic patients present with a spectrum of symptoms that vary in degree and severity from person to person. In older people and in the young the cardinal features of asthma, namely, wheezing and shortness of breath, may not be as apparent as in the rest of the population. Young children rarely wheeze with asthma (BTS SIGN 2003); rather they cough especially at night. Older people may not perceive their degree of airway restriction to be significant and accept chest tightness and shortness of breath as an 'ageing effect' (Chung 2002). The clinician should always consider the possibility of arriving at a diagnosis of asthma when discussing respiratory symptoms with these age groups. A diagnosis of asthma will only be made when the health professional is sensitive and alert to the possibility that the symptoms the patient is presenting may be a result of asthma.

Figure 2.2 outlines the diagnosis of asthma in adults.

RESPIRATORY FUNCTION TESTS

The obstruction of airflow in the respiratory airways can be measured by objective tests. The most common one used in the diagnosis of asthma is measurement of peak expiratory flow rate (PEFR) using a peak flow meter. (The technique used to perform this test is described in Chapter 8.) Asthma will reduce the force with which expired air can be exhaled from the airways, reducing the value read by the peak flow meter. The expected peak expiratory flow readings are dependent upon the patient's age, gender and height and based on those parameters it may be calculated. Comparison between the expected and actual readings are useful to provide a guide to assessing the degree of airflow obstruction. However as more data becomes available it is better to compare the PEFR readings with the patient's 'best ever' peak flow rate. Peak expiratory flow can help in the diagnosis of asthma. If the variability of PEFR is greater than 20% between the best (when patient is well) and the worst recording (when patient is experiencing asthma symptoms) then a diagnosis of asthma can be made.

Consider the diagnosis of asthma in patients with some or all of the following:

Symptoms
Episodic/variable
- wheeze
- shortness of breath
- chest tightness
- cough

Signs
- none *(common)*
- wheeze – diffuse, bilateral, expiratory *(± inspiratory)*
- tachypnoea

Helpful additional information
- Personal or family history of asthma or atopy *(eczema, allergic rhinitis)*
- History of worsening after use of aspirin/NSAID ingestion, use of β blockers *(including glaucoma drops)*
- Recognised triggers – pollens, dust, animals, exercise, viral infections, chemicals, irritants
- Pattern and severity of symptoms and exacerbations

Objective measurements
- >20% diurnal variation on ≥3 days in a week for two weeks on **PEF** diary
  or FEV_1 ≥15% (and 200 mL) increase after short acting $β_2$ agonist (e.g. salbutamol 400 mcg by pMDI + spacer or 2.5 mg by nebuliser)
  or FEV_1 ≥15% (and 200 mL) increase after trial of steroid tablets (prednisolone 30 mg/day for 14 days)
  or FEV_1 ≥15% decrease after six minutes of exercise (running)
- Histamine or methacholine challenge in difficult cases

Indication for referral for specialist opinion/ further investigation*
- Diagnosis unclear or in doubt
- Unexpected clinical findings *e.g. crackles, clubbing, cyanosis, heart failure*
- Spirometry or **PEFs** don't fit the clinical picture
- Suspected occupational asthma
- Persistent shortness of breath (not episodic, or without associated wheeze)
- Unilateral or fixed wheeze
- Stridor
- Persistent chest pain or atypical features
- Weight loss
- Persistent cough and/or sputum production
- Non-resolving pneumonia

Differential diagnoses include:
- Chronic obstructive pulmonary disease (COPD)
- cardiac disease
- tumour
  - laryngeal
  - tracheal
  - lung
- bronchiectasis
- foreign body
- interstitial lung disease
- pulmonary emboli
- aspiration
- vocal cord dysfunction
- hyperventilation

* Consider chest X-ray in any patient presenting atypically or with additional symptoms

Figure 2.2 Diagnosis of asthma in adults. With permission from BMJ Publishing Group (BTS/SIGN 2003).

Calculation of peak flow rate percentage variability (BTS 2003):

Highest peak flow rate = 400 L/min
Lowest peak flow rate = 300 L/min
Percentage PEF variability = $[^{(400 - 300)}/_{400}] \times 100\% = 25\%$

Peak flow diaries provide a valuable source of information to aid in the diagnosis and management of asthma. While there are slight variations from diary type to diary type they essentially all contain the following information.

The patient will record frequency of symptoms experienced, the frequency of medication used/required, and chart their peak expiratory flow readings a minimum of twice a day (morning and evening). Perusal of the peak flow diary can reveal vital clues to help in the management of the patient's asthma (see Fig. 2.3). This figure indicates three types of asthma status:

1. Well-controlled stable asthma.
2. Highly variable asthma which is a sign of a possible impending asthma attack.
3. Acute severe asthma which is probably life-threatening.

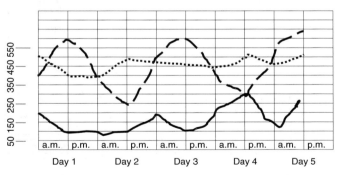

PEFR indicating acute severe asthma, requiring urgent intervention
PEFR indicating limited variation, stable asthma.
PEFR indicating large variability, severe asthma requiring intervention.

Figure 2.3 Peak flow diary. PEFR, peak expiratory flow rate.

The use of spirometry is also valuable in the diagnosis of asthma. Asthma will affect the forced expiratory volume (FEV_1) and reduce this figure from the expected value or, if the information is available, the patient's best (FEV_1). (The use of such data is discussed in Chapters 3 and 8.)

Medical history

Questionnaires have been designed to help the health professional to assess the patient's asthma (see Chapter 8). A useful brief questionnaire which has the ability to aid in the diagnosis of asthma is the 'International Union Against Tuberculosis and Lung Diseases' (IUATLD). This document includes the key questions:

- Have you had wheezing or whistling in your chest in the last 12 months?
- Have you had an attack of wheezing that came after stopping exercise?
- Have you had an attack of shortness of breath that came at any time of the day during a period when you were at rest?

These questions are similarly covered in ISAAC studies (International Study of Asthma and Allergies in Childhood Steering Committee). The questions are highly specific and indicate that the possibility of asthma must be considered if the answers affirm that any wheezing occurred during the periods of rest that followed exercise (Chung 2002).

Table 2.2 provides a list of conditions that should be covered in all new and repeat consultations with patients complaining of symptoms that could indicate a diagnosis of asthma.

Many health professionals will cover these key questions in consultations; it is important that the answers to these questions are clearly documented in the patient's medical records.

PHYSICAL EXAMINATION

If symptoms of airflow obstruction are present when the physical examination takes place this can aid in the diagnosis of asthma. Expiratory wheeze is a typical sign of airflow limitation, but it is not the most sensitive measure of this obstruction.

Table 2.2 Conditions to be considered when taking asthma history.

Symptoms	Cough, wheeze, shortness of breath, chest tightness and sputum production.
	Co-existence of other conditions associated with asthma: hay fever; rhinitis; sinusitis; atopic dermatitis (Chung 2002).
Pattern of symptoms	Perennial, seasonal, or perennial with seasonal exacerbations.
	Continuous, episodic or both.
	Onset, frequency and duration of symptoms.
	Diurnal variation of symptoms, nocturnal symptoms.
Precipitating/aggravating factors	Upper respiratory tract infections.
	Exposure to: viral allergens; housedust mites pollens; animal fur.
	Exposure to occupational chemicals or allergens.
	Exposure to irritants, e.g. tobacco smoke, air pollutants.
	Influence of emotional states and stress.
	Drugs, aspirin or non-steroidal anti-inflammatory agents, beta-blockers.
	Exercise.
	Weather changes.
History of disease development	Age of onset/diagnosis.
	Evolution of disease.
	Previous and current management of disease and response to treatment.
Profile of exacerbation	Speed of attack, management and outcome.
Social situation	Housing condition, exposure to allergens, animals at home, exposure to tobacco smoke, dampness, heating.
Severity of disease	Number of emergency treatments, including admissions to hospital, courses of oral steroids.
	Number of life-threatening episodes.
	Number of school/work days missed.
	Limitation of activity.
	Frequency of nocturnal awakenings.
	Effect on growth, behaviour, school or work achievements.
Impact of disease on family and relatives	
Family history: asthma or allergies in close relatives	

(Chung 2002, NRTC 1999).

Hyper-inflated chest, use of accessory muscles to breathe, inter-costal recession, cyanosis and drowsiness are clinical signs of respiratory distress and can indicate the presence of a severe asthma attack.

Asthma classification

Acute asthma can be classified into three groups as follows:

1. **Mild to moderate:** wheezing/coughing without severe distress; able to hold normal conversation; peak flow reading greater than 50% of best value.
2. **Moderate to severe:** wheezing/coughing with distress; talking in short sentences or phrases; peak flow reading less than 50% and some degree of oxygen de-saturation if measured by pulse oximetry. Obtained readings of between 90 and 95% saturation when measured by peripheral pulse oximetry.
3. **Severe, life-threatening:** severe respiratory distress; difficulty in talking; cyanosis; tired and confused; poor respiratory effort; few wheezes (silent chest) and weak breath sounds; tachypnoea; bradycardia; hypotension; peak flow less than 30% of predicated or best; oxygen saturations less than 90% when measured by peripheral pulse oximetry (BTS SIGN 2003, Chung 2002).

A note of caution should be considered in the diagnosis of asthma; please refer back to Figure 2.2. Not all wheeze is caused by asthma. For example, in children the inhalation of a foreign body can produce symptoms comparable to asthma; a cancerous tumour within the respiratory airways can also replicate asthma symptoms.

Asthma prevalence

There is a wide geographical variation in the prevalence of physician-diagnosed asthma in Europe (Chung 2002, Rabe *et al*. 2000). The highest prevalence is within the UK, and some areas of France. General Practitioners are becoming more aware of asthma and its symptoms, particularly within children. However, even allowing for this increase in symptom detection, the increase in asthma cannot be purely placed upon an increased knowledge base of GPs (Chung 2002).

Asthma morbidity can be devastating, not just for those with asthma, but also for their families and friends. Asthma morbidity includes: nocturnal wheezing; coughing; an inability to participate fully in everyday activities; days absent from school/ work and therefore an increased risk of under-achieving. Asthma symptoms are frequently accepted by those with asthma, and perceived by them as being something that they have to 'put up' with. In a survey of 2000 secondary school aged children with asthma, over a third of them had been woken up more than once in the preceding five days due to their asthma (Francis 2001). This is further confirmed by the statistic that over a third of children with asthma miss more than one week from school per year due to their asthma, with up to 49% of adults similarly reporting that they were not able to attend work in the preceding year on at least one occasion.

Rabe *et al.* in 2000 conducted a telephone survey across Europe. This survey revealed some concerning information. The results revealed that:

- 30% of adult patients with asthma said their sleep had been disturbed in the past week due to their asthma.
- 63% had some reduction in daily activities.
- 61% had experienced severe episodes of coughing, wheezing chest tightness.
- 30% had to access emergency health care.
- 41% of these patients reported that they were treated with medication to reduce and control their asthma symptoms.

Obviously this information indicates that people are coping with a high degree of asthma symptoms, which could be greatly reduced if the patient seeks help and shows compliance with the correct and appropriate asthma treatment.

MORTALITY FROM ASTHMA

Asthma mortality is generally low throughout the world in comparison with other diseases such as coronary heart disease or cancer. However, for a disease that has a number of treatment options, the mortality rate is still unacceptably high in England and Wales. In 1997 asthma was given as the cause of one death in forty, with 1584 deaths due to asthma out of the total 63 000 deaths in England and Wales.

The decrease in asthma mortality in England and Wales has occurred throughout the age range 2–74 years of age; however in the older population (greater than 75 years of age) asthma mortality is increasing. There are probably many reasons for this, but it is important in establishing the cause of death that the difficult differential diagnoses of asthma against COPD should have been carefully considered in those patients that had respiratory symptoms (Francis 2004).

MANAGEMENT OF ASTHMA

Pharmacological management

The aims of pharmacological management are to control symptoms including nocturnal symptoms and exercise induced asthma; to prevent exacerbations and achieve the greatest level of respiratory functioning with the minimal level of side effects (BTS SIGN 2003).

The British Thoracic Society (2003) guidelines follow a stepwise approach to the treatment of asthma, and recommend that the health professional commences asthma medication at a level most likely to achieve the aims given above. The overall objective is to achieve early and effective control of asthma and maintain flexible control by stepping up or down with the therapy as necessary. This stepwise approach to asthma management is illustrated in Fig. 2.4.

Synopsis of BTS (2003) asthma guidelines

STEP ONE: Short-acting bronchodilators (such as β_2 agonists, inhaled ipratropium bromide) should be prescribed as symptomatic relief for all patients with symptomatic asthma. (For mode of action of these medications see Chapter 3.) The frequency with which the patient makes use of such short-acting bronchodilators provides some measure of the severity of the

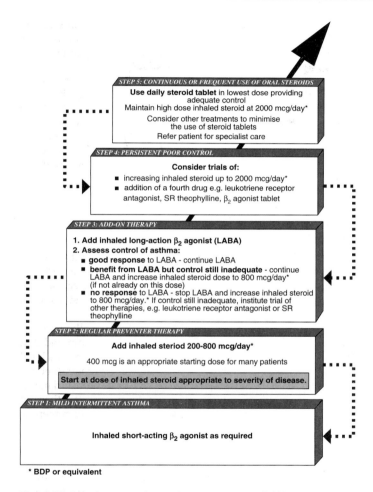

STEP 5: CONTINUOUS OR FREQUENT USE OF ORAL STEROIDS

Use daily steroid tablet in lowest dose providing adequate control

Maintain high dose inhaled steroid at 2000 mcg/day*

Consider other treatments to minimise the use of steroid tablets

Refer patient for specialist care

STEP 4: PERSISTENT POOR CONTROL

Consider trials of:

- increasing inhaled steroid up to 2000 mcg/day*
- addition of a fourth drug e.g. leukotriene receptor antagonist, SR theophylline, β_2 agonist tablet

STEP 3: ADD-ON THERAPY

1. Add inhaled long-action β_2 agonist (LABA)
2. Assess control of asthma:
   - **good response** to LABA - continue LABA
   - **benefit from LABA but control still inadequate** - continue LABA and increase inhaled steroid dose to 800 mcg/day* (if not already on this dose)
   - **no response** to LABA - stop LABA and increase inhaled steroid to 800 mcg/day.* If control still inadequate, institute trial of other therapies, e.g. leukotriene receptor antagonist or SR theophylline

STEP 2: REGULAR PREVENTER THERAPY

Add inhaled steriod 200-800 mcg/day*

400 mcg is an appropriate starting dose for many patients

Start at dose of inhaled steroid appropriate to severity of disease.

STEP 1: MILD INTERMITTENT ASTHMA

Inhaled short-acting β_2 agonist as required

* BDP or equivalent

Figure 2.4 Stepwise approach to asthma management. With permission BMJ Publishing Group (BTS/SIGN 2003).

patient's asthma and/or their compliance with other medication.

STEP TWO: Introduction of preventer therapy. Inhaled steroids are the recommended preventer therapy for both adults and children. They should be prescribed for patients with recent exacerbations, nocturnal asthma or impaired lung function or those using inhaled β_2 agonists more than once a day. Other preventer therapies are not the first choice medication at 'Step Two'; however if there are clinical or patient-centred reasons for not prescribing inhaled steroids then sodium cromoglycate, leukotriene receptor antagonists, or theophylline may be prescribed.

STEP THREE: Add-on therapy. Before commencing this step it is important that all other parameters must be checked: such as patient compliance with medication; ability to use inhalers appropriately and avoidance of trigger factors. (Chapter 4 discusses inhaler medication in greater detail.) Add-on therapy includes long-acting β_2 agonists, increased inhaled steroid dose, leukotriene receptor antagonist, theophylline.

STEP FOUR: Indicated by poor control of asthma symptoms. In this case addition of a fourth drug is recommended.

STEP FIVE: As above with the addition of continuous or frequently administered oral steroids. In this case regular monitoring of the whole physiological functioning of the patient is recommended since oral steroids have shown significant side effects associated with them. This monitoring includes growth monitoring in children and observation for onset of diabetes, osteoporosis, hypertension and cataract development.

Non-pharmacological management of asthma

Precipitating factors that can trigger an asthma attack/exacerbate chronic asthma

Exercise can precipitate airway narrowing in most asthmatic patients (Rees & Kanabar 2000). The response of patients to exercise is important as a diagnostic tool in those cases where asthma is suspected. Undertaking vigorous exercise can induce asthma symptoms which when they occur in a clinical situation can be monitored and documented. Exercise-induced asthma is a significant problem for children at school and the current advice is to take prophylactically β_2 agonists some 5–15 minutes prior the event and then repeat the medication when required to reduce any asthma symptoms that appear.

Allergens can trigger asthma attacks and increase asthma morbidity. They should be considered in any review of the management of the patient's asthma. The identification of putative allergens should be attempted by taking a detailed medical history, and carrying out allergy testing when possible. Following the identification of any allergens that trigger the patient's asthma the management plan should promote methods to remove, minimise or avoid specific allergens. Common allergens are housedust mites, animal dander, pollens and spores.

Breastfeeding exclusively for the first four or more months of a baby's life has been shown to reduce the chance of an incidence of asthma occurring after the child reaches the age of six. This effect is more significant in those children who have a high degree of family history of atopy. The hygiene hypothesis suggests that some exposure in early life (when an infant) to microbial products (allergens) will, in later life, reduce any tendency to produce an acute allergic response to those allergens. The immune response may be somehow 'attenuated' and fail to trigger the onset of an asthmatic episode (Strachan 2000).

Occupational asthma is a significant problem; this form of the 'trauma' is defined as asthma that arises in adults who have not previously had asthma, or have their asthma exacerbated by exposure to an allergen at work. It is one of the most frequently reported respiratory diseases in the UK and many other countries. It is estimated that each year in the UK, 1500–3000 people develop asthma (new cases) as a direct response to their work environment (BOHRF 2004). This type of asthma is preventable. Its elimination is dependent upon the establishment of effective controls that will result in a reduction of the risks that result from the workers' exposure to respiratory sensitisers present in their workplace.

As it is with any other respiratory disease, tobacco smoking is detrimental to the management of asthma. Despite the evidence that has been available for decades that 'passive smoking' contributes to the severity of childhood asthma, health workers should still seek every opportunity to encourage parents to cease smoking (BTS SIGN 2003).

Complementary therapies for the management of asthma are considered in detail in the BTS 2003 guidelines, and these include acupuncture, homeopathy, hypnosis, and breathing exercises. It is worth referring to this publication for further information on these topics.

Management of acute severe asthma

Investigation into 200 asthma deaths in England and Wales reveals that many of these patients had 'histories' which probably contributed directly to their deaths. These earlier indications could be shown to be associated with: the disease itself; its medical management; or the patient's own behaviour. Most deaths occurred prior to admission to hospital (Wareham *et al.* 1993, Mohan *et al.* 1996, Burr *et al.* 1999). The majority of those who died had chronically severe asthma; in only a minority of cases did the attack occur suddenly in a patient with mild or moderate disease symptoms.

The risk factors for developing near fatal or fatal asthma are multifactorial and include the following:

- Previous near fatal asthma (requiring ventilation, and or developing respiratory acidosis).
- Previous admission to hospital for asthma especially within the last year.
- Requiring three or more classes of asthma medication.
- Brittle asthma.
- Non-compliance with medication.
- Failure to attend medical appointments.
- Denial.
- Psychological problems.
- Severe stress (BTS SIGN 2003).

It has been stated that most severe asthma attacks that require hospital admission develop over a period of six or more hours. It should thus be possible to intervene appropriately and commence action that will either eliminate the need for hospital admission or greatly reduce the severity of the asthma attack (Kolbe *et al*. 1998, Woodruff *et al*. 1998, Kolbe *et al*. 2000).

All health professionals should be aware of the symptoms of respiratory distress and the possible implications that asthma symptoms can have for the patient (BTS SIGN 2003). In cases of asthma patients complaining of respiratory symptoms these should be assessed against the criteria produced by the BTS and summarised under 'Synopsis of BTS (2003) asthma guidelines'.

Hospital referral is essential for any patients with features of acute severe or life-threatening asthma.

Treatment of acute severe asthma in adults

These patients will have many if not all of the signs and symptoms of respiratory distress. This includes: tachypnoea; using accessory muscles to aid in breathing; tachycardia; cyanosis; peripheral pulse oximetry reading less than 90%; unable to talk in complete sentences; eat or drink; wheezing or the more sinister situation the 'silent chest' (see Chapters 5 and 8). The priority in these circumstances is to reduce the respiratory distress and relieve the hypoxaemia. Patient assessment is always undertaken and the severity of the patient's asthma assessed immediately upon arrival in the hospital environment. However in asthma crisis it would not be appropriate to utilise the whole respiratory assessment proforma discussed in Chapter 8 and waste time in considering the patient's asthma-related quality of life. Judicious assessment appropriately timed and correctly carried out will provide valuable and succinct information concerning the degree of asthma severity. Health status and related information can be assessed after the acute crisis is resolved.

Dyspnoea (difficulty in breathing) is very, very frightening and anyone who experiences this should be constantly reassured and kept fully informed of their condition. Any improvement in symptoms should always be noted and reported back to the patients who may be too exhausted to observe this improvement for themselves.

The management of acute severe asthma is clearly outlined in the 2003 BTS asthma guidelines; however many hospitals will also have their own proforma or protocols that are followed. In general the use of guidelines to aid in decision-making concerning asthma management is beneficial to patient care.

Oxygen therapy

These patients will be hypoxaemic (see Chapter 5) and require oxygen therapy; this should be high flow and high concentration oxygen therapy, sufficient to maintain peripheral pulse oximetry readings above 92%. The selection of facemask is important to ensure that the patient will have maximum delivery of oxygen and this is discussed in greater detail in Chapter 5.

β_2 agonists should be administered as soon as possible to reduce the bronchospasm responsible in part for the airflow obstruction. In practice it is found that in cases of acute severe asthma it is usually difficult to administer this medication via a pressured metered dose inhaler (pMDI) used in conjunction with a large volume spacer; the patient is usually too unwell to co-operate. However, if the patient is able to tolerate this route of drug administration and does not have the features of life-threatening asthma, it can be shown to be as clinically effective as the results using a nebuliser to deliver this therapy (see Chapter 8). In acute severe asthma in which the patient is hypoxaemic, it is necessary to continue to administer β_2 agonists via an oxygen-driven nebuliser in order to reduce the risk of further desaturation of the patient (BTS SIGN 2003).

This medication should be repeated at 15–30 minute intervals; continuous nebulisation therapy is reserved for asthma that does not appear to respond to the bolus nebulisation delivery.

Steroid therapy

Steroid therapy should be commenced as soon as possible; if the patient can swallow and retain oral steroid medication (prednisolone) this is the route of choice for delivery. Oral steroid medication is as effective as intravenous steroid therapy (Rowe *et al*. 2001). However in acute severe asthma many patients may not be able to tolerate oral medication; in this instance intravenous hydrocortisone is administered. As soon as the patient can tolerate oral medication intravenous steroid therapy should be discontinued and medication switched to oral therapy.

Steroid medication (40–50 mg prednisolone) should continue daily for at least five days or until recovery (BTS SIGN 2003). Issues surrounding tapering down of oral steroid medication in order to cease the medication are not of relevance unless:

- the oral steroid medication dose is exceptionally high;
- the patient already has regular oral steroid medication;
- or the duration of treatment has been longer than three weeks.

Ipratropium bromide

The combination of nebulised ipratropium bromide with a β_2 agonist has been proven to significantly increase the bronchodilation effect in acute severe asthma. Its use should be considered in acute severe asthma, although it may not be required in the less severe asthma attacks.

Intravenous aminophylline

The 2003 BTS asthma guidelines state that the use of intravenous aminophylline is unlikely to have a positive benefit upon the bronchoconstriction of acute severe asthma. The guidelines suggest that the significant side effects of aminophylline such as palpitations, arrhythmias and vomiting will be more detrimental to the patient than its questionable positive benefits. Its narrow therapeutic index makes the use of aminophylline a matter for careful decision and if it is commenced the aminophylline levels in blood plasma should be checked daily.

Intravenous fluids may be necessary to compensate for any electrolyte imbalances or fluid imbalance that may be occurring due to vomiting and increased respiration rate. It is always wise to have intravenous access in those patients with acute severe asthma, since this condition can deteriorate to 'life-threatening asthma' and may require full resuscitation.

Referral to intensive care should be considered in all situations in which ventilatory support is being considered for the patient, or for those who are failing to respond to treatment. Criteria for this referral are quite clearly expressed in the 2003 asthma guidelines.

Management following the acute episode

Following recovery from an acute episode of asthma 'discharge home' is considered when:

- the peak expiratory flow rates are consistently more than 75% of best or predicted;
- there are no clinical signs of respiratory failure;
- and the oxygen saturation remains above 95% as measure by peripheral pulse oximetry when breathing room air (Chung 2002).

Even though all the criteria given above are satisfied, this is not sufficient on its own to warrant a decision to 'discharge home'. It is the responsibility of the health professionals caring for these patients to ensure that the risk factors that exist for a subsequent severe asthma attack are reduced. This includes assessment and identification, where possible, of the precipitating factors that induced the recent attack. An attempt to address these issues should be made to obtain a reduction in the number of further asthmatic attacks. Upon discharge home the patient should be asked to have their asthma reviewed by their primary care practice and for it to be undertaken by either the GP or practice nurse. This establishes the follow up care necessary for the patient and reaffirms the importance of continuous care management of a chronic disease. The 2003 BTS asthma guidelines suggest that this follow-up should be within two days following discharge; however this is often not possible if the patient is discharged on a Friday. The discharge timing from acute hospital-based care should be considered in relation to the availability of primary health care support and the need for relevant patient education.

This information may be gathered over a significant time period, and does not need to be extracted from a patient by a

Table 2.3 Asthmatic patient's own knowledge.

A full comprehensive detailed assessment of the patient's asthma should address:
Patient's knowledge and understanding of their own asthma. Patient's own self-management strategies used when their asthma is deteriorating. Asthma health status and morbidity. Compliance with medication. Inhaler technique. Identification of the precipitating factors which may include triggers to patient's asthma such as pollen, upper respiratory tract infections, animal dander.

long interrogation! However it is important that the information is obtained, since one of the major risk factors for fatal or near fatal asthma attack is the occurrence of an acute severe asthma attack in the preceding year. It is impossible to remove this risk factor, but all other risk factors must be addressed in order to minimise the possibility of a second severe or life-threatening attack.

The health professional should work in partnership with the patient who has asthma and by forming a therapeutic relationship become able to exchange information and ideas freely (Table 2.3). Issues that are raised in discussions about compliance with medication, ability to use inhaler devices and knowledge concerning medication regime can thus be resolved in an appropriate manner and at a suitable pace for the patient.

There is an art to giving information; it should be timed appropriately for the patient and be at a suitable level for their existing knowledge base. Factors such as: ability to comprehend verbal information; ability to understand English; ability to concentrate for a period of time sufficient for information to be given all need to be considered by the health care professional. Caress *et al.* (2003) suggest that so important is this information-giving that it needs significant consideration by the health professional prior to its commencement.

A synopsis of the factors and subjects that should be addressed are outlined in Tables 2.4 and 2.5.

Table 2.4 Key considerations in information giving.

Timing (when to give the information)
Volume (how much to give)
Topic (what to give)
Process (how to give the information)
Format (what medium to use)
Special circumstances (e.g. low literacy, children, ethnic minorities)

With permission from Caress *et al.* (2003) Information giving in asthma care. *Airways Journal* 1: 77–81.

Table 2.5 Information topics to address with patients – advice from the new BTS/SIGN guideline on asthma management.

Nature of disease
Nature of treatment
Areas where patient most wants treatment to have an effect
How to use treatment
Self-monitoring/self-assessment skills
Negotiation of asthma action plan in light of identified patient goals
Recognition and management of acute exacerbations
Appropriate allergen or trigger avoidance

With permission from Caress *et al.* (2003) Information giving in asthma care. *Airways Journal* 1: 77–81.

Asthma self-management by the patient has been proven to reduce the number of school and work days lost due to asthma and results in fewer visits to emergency departments (BTS SIGN 2003). The patients are especially directed towards the implementation and use of personalised action plans; the stratagem appears to work for children and adults in all health care environments and can be issued by any health care professional (Gallefoss & Bakke 2000, Gibson *et al*. 2001). Action plans identify features that the patient can measure, such as peak expiratory flow rate or the symptoms that the patient experiences and recognises as indicators of a change in the patient's asthma. The action plans then provide information that allows the patient to manage their own asthma, such as seeking urgent medical advice when peak expiratory flow rate falls below a patient-centred fixed point, or commencing oral steroid medication. It is important that these action plans are written in conjunction with the patient. Both the health carer and the patient should have agreed the primary goals and the information contained within them, otherwise they are unlikely to be used by the patient and are thus rendered useless.

Management of asthma in primary care

The routine management of asthma is based within primary care; many general practices will have GPs and practice nurses with specific training in asthma care and management. It would appear to make little difference which one performs the routine care of the asthmatic patient, whether it is the GP, pharmacist or practice nurse as long as the review process is undertaken (Watanabe *et al.* 1998). However some observational studies have suggested that the practice nurse with a suitable asthma qualification is perhaps best able to provide this type of care (Dickenson *et al.* 1997, Lindberg *et al.* 1999).

Setting up asthma reviews and a 'call and recall' programme requires some consideration by all within the general practice. It should be carefully considered and evaluated once the initial set up is complete. A brief resume for the setting up of an asthma programme is provided in Table 2.6.

General practices should keep records of those patients with diagnosed asthma and should at regular intervals call them into

Table 2.6 Checklist 1. Setting up a structured asthma programme.

Investigate the availability of resources. This should include written asthma action plans and information leaflets, etc. Non-promotional material is available form the National Asthma Campaign (www.asthma.org.uk)

Seek consensus opinion to ensure all members of the team are giving consistent advice.

Discuss practical aspects of implementation. Points to consider will include: which patients to target; whether education is to be integrated into usual care and delivered in one-to-one consultations or delivered to groups of patients.

Tailor the education and advice to the individual needs of the patient, respecting differing ambitions, wishes for autonomy and their age.

Reproduced with permission from British Guidelines on the Management of Asthma (2003) *Thorax* **58** (Suppl. 1): i1–i94 BMJ Publishing.

Table 2.7 Checklist 2. Suggested content for an educational programme/ discussion.

This checklist is intended as an example that health professionals should adapt to meet the needs of individual patients and/or carers. The purpose of education is to empower patients and/or carers to undertake self-management more appropriately and effectively. Information given should be tailored to an individual's social, emotional and disease status and age. Different approaches are needed for different ages.

- Nature of disease.
- Nature of treatment.
- Identify areas where patient most wants treatment to have effect.
- How to use treatment.
- Development of self-monitoring/self-assessment skills.
- Negotiation of the asthma action plan in light of identified patient goals.
- Recognition and management of acute exacerbations.
- Appropriate allergen or trigger avoidance.

Reproduced with permission from British Guideline on the Management of Asthma (2003) *Thorax* **58** (Suppl. 1): i1–i94 BMJ Publishing.

Table 2.8 Asthma symptom level.

- Symptom level and incidence of any recent asthma exacerbation including necessity for short course oral steroids, emergency visits to hospital or GP. (Always ask, since the patient may have been away from their own home when requiring urgent medical attention and the paperwork may not yet have caught up with their own notes in the medical practice!)
- Smoking history.
- Use of asthma action plans/requirement for an update.
- Asthma-related issues that patient would like to discuss.
- Compliance with medication and inhaler technique.
- Giving of written or verbal information to aid the patient in recalling the interview. All the 'information giving' should be in accordance with standard National Guidelines such as the British Guideline on the Management of Asthma (2003).

the practice for an asthma review. This review should broadly follow the following guidelines, however it is important that it is tailored for the individual patient and their concerns. Patient queries should always be prioritised and addressed; it is not good practice to ignore these in an attempt to tick all the relevant documentation in an asthma review.

Topics that should be addressed in an asthma review include all those items listed in Tables 2.6 and 2.7 together with the factors in Table 2.8.

The use of detailed review and assessment has been proven to reduce school or work absence due to asthma, reduce asthma exacerbation rate and improve symptom control (Charlton *et al.* 1991, Droogan & Bannigan 1997, Hoskins *et al.* 1999). It is thus a very important component in the continued management and reduction of asthma symptoms.

Case study: John Adams, Part 1

John Adams (22 years of age) arrived in the accident and emergency department with obvious respiratory distress. He was driven in by his flatmate from university. Initial assessment revealed the following: his respiration rate was 32 breaths per minute; using all his accessory muscles to breathe; unable to talk due to his dyspnoea; heart rate 134 beats per minute; peripheral pulse oximetry revealed saturations of 86% and he was visibly cyanosed. No obvious indication of chest trauma, or cardiac event, but John's friend from university stated that John used a blue inhaler at times.

Initial therapy as follows: high flow oxygen delivered via an oxygen mask capable of delivering high concentration oxygen; nebulised (oxygen-driven) salbutamol and ipratropium bromide. Intravenous fluids and hydrocortisone was prescribed and a chest X-ray (CXR) taken to ensure that some other causes of respiratory distress could be eliminated. The nebulised salbutamol was repeated every 15 minutes for an hour and an improvement in John's condition was noted.

Physical examination of John and his CXR indicated that he did not have a chest infection and the most likely cause of his dyspnoea was an exacerbation of his asthma. John's response to therapy was in accordance with the BTS (2003) British Guideline on the Management of Asthma, and would indicate that John was experiencing an acute/severe asthma exacerbation.

ROUTINE ASTHMA PHARMACOLOGICAL THERAPY

Bronchodilator medication

These medications have an anti-bronchoconstrictor effect and will cause an immediate reversal of airway obstruction in asthma mainly as a result of their primary effect upon airway smooth muscle.

There are three types of bronchodilator:

1. **β_2 adrenergic agonists** (e.g. salbutamol, terbutaline are short-acting; longer acting drugs includes salmeterol and formoterol).
2. **Methylxanthines** (e.g. aminophylline and theophylline).
3. **Anticholinergic drugs** (e.g. ipratropium bromide).

β_2 adrenergic agonists

β_2 adrenergic agonists are usually considered to be the most effective types of bronchodilators available. They stimulate the β_2 receptors located within the airways and cause relaxation of airway smooth muscle. They have limited side effects associated with their use. However they can cause muscle tremor, tachycardia and palpitations. Method of delivery of these medications is usually via the inhaled route, and although they can be administered intravenously this is rarely carried out. The choice of inhaler device and its use depends upon many factors such as patient ability to use the inhaler, patient choice and in some cases cost (see Chapter 4 for further discussion).

Methylxanthines

Theophylline has been used for the treatment of asthma since 1930 (Chung 2002). It is available as a slow release preparation and is a known bronchodilator. However although its precise mode of action is unclear, it is postulated that it effects its therapeutic role by modulating the intracellular concentrations of cAMP, even though it is known that in therapeutic concentrations this putative effect is weak. It may have an effect upon the T-cells by inhibiting the airway leakage of plasma and associated oedema (Chung 2002). Although theophylline is used in clinical practice, it does however have serious side effects associated with its use, such as cardiac arrhythmias and epileptic fits. Thus those patients receiving theophylline therapy require that the drug's plasma concentration be closely monitored.

Anticholinergic drugs

Anticholinergics antagonise the muscarinic receptors of the airway and thus inhibit bronchoconstriction caused by the stimulation of cholinergic nerves. These medicines may thus be more effective when used as protection against stimuli such as dust or cold air, which can cause bronchoconstriction in susceptible individuals. Mode of delivery is usually the inhaled route (see Chapter 4).

Inhaled corticosteroids
(e.g. budesonide, betamethasone, fluticasone)

These are recommended as a first-line therapy for the treatment of asthma (BTS SIGN 2003). It is suggested that the initial dose be sufficient to achieve control of asthma symptoms and gain compliance with the medication regimen. Once control has been achieved all medication should be reviewed and then titrated (usually downwards) to a maintenance dose. They are usually administered twice a day although once daily preparations are available. Choice of inhaler device depends upon inhaled steroid prescribed, patient ability to use inhaler, and other factors (see Chapter 4).

Corticosteroids reduce the inflammatory process in asthma; these drugs have a direct effect upon many of the cells and signalling pathways involved. The corticosteroids are effective in reducing the numbers of mast cells, eosinophils and lymphocytes within the airways as well as producing a reduction of mediators associated with airway inflammation. Clinically they will improve the lung function of those with asthma, reducing not only the use of symptomatic relief medication, but also diminishing exacerbation and the need for oral steroid therapy.

Side effects from steroids are related to the route of delivery and the concentration absorbed by the body.

Inhaled corticosteroids in high doses will cause adrenal suppression, growth suppression, bruising, reduced bone density and cataracts, and can cause local effects such as dysphoria and oral candidiasis.

Oral steroid therapy has a greater frequency of side effects and these include: adrenal growth suppression, bruising, osteoporosis, growth suppression, cataracts, glaucoma, and other metabolic disturbances.

Oral steroid therapy is reserved for the treatment of acute exacerbations of asthma or for the treatment of difficult to control 'brittle' asthma. It is prescribed in the attempt to gain rapid control of the inflammation processes occurring in the airway.

Sodium cromoglycate is an inhaled medication used to reduce the inflammation characteristic of asthma. It acts upon mast cells and reduces the production of IgE and the histamine release that IgE triggers. These changes are followed by a decreased amount of inflammation within the airways. It is more effective in atopic individuals and can protect well against seasonal exacerbations of asthma.

Side effects are limited and are usually transient. Any coughing upon administration of medication can be prevented by prior inhalation of β_2 agonist.

Anti-leukotrienes (montelukast, zafirlukast)
Leukotriene receptor antagonists inhibit the effects of cysteinyl-leukotrienes released during an asthma attack. These cysteinyl-leukotrienes are released from inflammatory cells in the airway and cause bronchoconstriction and oedema and stimulate mucus secretion. Thus the inhibition of these adverse reactions will greatly reduce the airflow obstruction associated with asthma.

Clinically they are recommended in the 2003 BTS asthma guidelines as an 'add-on therapy' after the commencement of inhaled steroids. They are usually well tolerated, although their side effects can include headaches, nausea and vomiting, skin rashes, and gastrointestinal upsets.

Other treatments

Antihistamines are not recommended for the treatment of asthma, although if accompanying rhinitis exits then this should be treated with non-sedating antihistamines.

Immunotherapy

Desensitisation therapy can be beneficial in cases of life-threatening anaphylactic allergic reactions, e.g. to bee and wasp stings. It is also useful in reducing sensitivity to grass pollens however in many cases of asthma it is not an appropriate treatment.

Case study: John Adams, Part 2

John spent five days in hospital. During his first day he remained acutely unwell; he required repeated 15-minute nebulisations of salbutamol and ipratropium bromide and high concentration of humidified oxygen. His peripheral pulse oximetry improved with this therapy to 92% and his arterial blood gas analysis revealed hypoxaemia but no hypercapnia or acidosis.

Prior to his discharge John wished to discuss his asthma with every health professional who would listen, since he was quite distressed by his severe asthma attack. This incentive from John helped the respiratory nurse specialist to discuss and identify the possible causes of John's severe asthma attack and elucidate some self-management strategies to enable John to manage his own asthma. It became apparent that since attending university John had ceased to take his regular preventative therapy for his asthma and only routinely used his reliever medication. He had noticed an increased need for his reliever medication and had merely though it was due to exam stress.

Detailed review of John's asthma-related morbidity revealed that every day for several months he was wheezy;

Continued

> he could not walk up two flights of stairs without requiring his reliever medication and would wake up at night coughing. He was experiencing stress at present with his university examinations and had just broken up with his long-term girlfriend.
>
> John was sent home with a detailed asthma management plan, based upon his symptoms and peak expiratory flow rate. He was recommenced on preventative inhaled therapy and taught how to use his inhalers correctly. He was required to continue with oral steroid therapy for another five days and was requested to see his own general practitioner/practice nurse within the next two days to review his asthma upon discharge.
>
> An outpatient appointment was made for John one month following his discharge home to review his asthma management.

Alternative methods

Those who seek alternative therapies often report significant benefits from these treatments (Markham & Wilkinson 2004); however at present there is little rigorous evidence to substantiate their claims. The use of this method of asthma treatment is of 'patient preference' and it is important that the health professional responsible for the conventional management of the patient's asthma provides adequate information for the patient to be able to manage their asthma appropriately.

New approaches to pharmacologic asthma treatment

The cellular milieu of airway inflammation is the target for the future asthma therapies. It is possible that the inhibition of specific pathways in asthma inflammation will be targeted. The use of monoclonal antibodies will be able to hinder the transcription of specific genes and thus inhibit identified cellular pathways in the inflammation response of airways (Rambasek *et al.* 2004). The days of 'generic medication' treating the inflammation process of the airways by virtue of their route of inhaled deposition are numbered (Storms 2003). It may eventually be possible to have specific 'patient unique medication' that completely controls their asthma, eliminating all symptoms of the disease.

The reduction of the allergic response that triggers atopic asthma is also under scrutiny: if the allergy that triggers asthma attacks can be removed then the need for anti-asthma medication is removed.

The developments in the treatment of asthma that have occurred in the last decade have been exciting; the future decade may be even more so.

SUMMARY

❏ Asthma is a common disease throughout the world and has a high incidence in the UK.
❏ Asthma has a high level of morbidity associated with it and is responsible on average for over 1500 deaths a year in the UK.
❏ Asthma management within the UK is based upon the reduction of symptoms and maintaining patient quality of life.
❏ The BTS (2003) British Guidelines on the Management of Asthma are recommended to be followed in the treatment of asthma in the UK.
❏ Acute severe asthma can be life-threatening and its management is usually within a hospital environment.
❏ Routine management of asthma is carried out in primary care.
❏ Patient information and self-management strategies are essential in empowering those with asthma to control their own disease.
❏ Asthma pharmacological treatment is based upon relieving the bronchoconstriction and inflammation associated with the airways of asthmatic patients.

REFERENCES

Anderson HR, Butland BK, Strachan DP (1994) Trends in prevalence and severity of childhood asthma. *BMJ* **308**: 1600–1604.

Ayres JG, Miles JF, Barnes PJ (1998) Brittle asthma. *Thorax* **53**: 315–321.

Bourke SJ, (2003) *Lecture notes on respiratory medicine*, 6th edn. Blackwell Publishing, Oxford.

Brand PL, Postma DS, Kerstjens HA, Koete GH (1991) Relationship of airway hyperresponsiveness to respiratory symptoms and diurnal peak flow variation in patients with obstructive lung disease. *American Review of Respiratory Disease* **143**: 916–921.

British Occupational Health Research Foundation (BOHRF) (2004) *Guidelines for the prevention, identification and management of occupational asthma: evidence review and recommendations* September: 1–37.

British Thoracic Society, National Asthma Campaign, Royal College of Physicians of London in association with the General Practitioner in Asthma Group *et al.* (1997) The British Guidelines on Asthma Management: 1995 review and position statement. *Thorax* **52** (Suppl. 1): S1–S21.

BTS/SIGN (2003) British Guideline on the Management of Asthma. *Thorax* **53** (Suppl. 1): i1–i94.

Bucknall CE, Slack R, Godley CC *et al.* (1999) Scottish confidential inquiry into asthma deaths (SCIAD). *Thorax* **54**: 978–984.

Burr ML, Davies BH, Hoare A *et al.* (1999) A confidential inquiry into asthma deaths in Wales. *Thorax* **54**: 985–989.

Caress AL, Beaver K, Woodcock A, Luker K (2003) Information giving in asthma care. *Airways Journal* **1**: 77–81.

Charlton I, Charlton G, Broomfield J *et al.* (1991) Audit of the effect of a nurse run asthma clinic on the workload and patient morbidity in a general practice. *British Journal of General Practice* **41**: 227–231.

Chee CB, Wang SY, Poh SC (1996) Department audit of inpatient management of asthma. *Singapore Medicine Journal* **37** (4): 370–373.

Chung KF (2002) *Clinicians' guide to asthma*. Arnold, London.

Ciba Guest Symposium (1959) Terminology, definition and classification of chronic pulmonary emphysema and related conditions. *Thorax* **14**: 286–299.

Dickenson J, Hutton S, Atkin A *et al.* (1997) Reducing asthma morbidity in the community: the effect of a targeted nurse run asthma clinic in an English general practice. *Respiratory Medicine* **91**: 634–640.

Droogan J, Bannigan K (1997) Organisation of asthma care: what difference does it make? *Nursing Times* **93**: 45–46.

Francis C (2001) School clinics for adolescents with asthma. *Professional Nurse* **16** (8): 1281–1284.

Francis C (2004) Asthma and older people: improving nursing care. *Nursing Older People* **16** (4): 22–27.

Gallefoss F, Bakke PS (2000) Impact of patient education and self management on morbidity in asthmatics and patients with chronic obstructive disease. *Respiratory Medicine* **94**: 279–287.

Gibson PG, Coughlan J, Wilson AJ *et al.* (2001) Self management and regular practitioner review for adults with asthma (Cochrane review). In: *Cochrane Library Issue 3.* Oxford.

Global Initiative for Asthma (GINA) (1995) Global strategy for asthma management and prevention. *NHLBI/WHO workshop report.* NIH publication No. 95-3659: 1–46.

Hoskins G, Neville RG, Smith B *et al.* (1999) The link between nurse training and asthma outcomes. *British Journal of Community Nursing* 4: 222–228.

International Consensus Report on the Diagnosis and Management of Asthma (1992) *Clinical Expiration Allergy* **22** Suppl. 1.

International Study of Asthma and Allergies in Childhood (ISAAC) Steering Committee (1998) Worldwide variation in prevalence of symptoms of asthma, allergic rhinoconjunctivitis and atopic eczema. *Lancet* **351**: 1225–1232.

Kolbe J, Fergusson W, Garrett J (1998) Rapid onset asthma: a severe but uncommon manifestation. *Thorax* **53**: 241–247.

Kolbe J, Fergusson W, Vamos M *et al.* (2000) Case control study of severe life threatening asthma (SLTA) in adults, demographics, health care and management of acute attack. *Thorax* **55**: 1007–1015.

Lewis S, Butland B, Strachan D *et al.* (1996) Study of the aetiology of wheezing illness at age 16 in two national British born cohorts. *Thorax* **51**: 6706–6710.

Lindberg M, Ahlner J, Moller M *et al.* (1999) Asthma nurse practice – a resource effective approach in asthma management. *Respiratory Medicine* **93**: 584–588.

Markham AW, Wilkinson JM (2004) Complementary and alternative medicines (CAM) in the management of asthma: an examination of the evidence. *Journal of Asthma* **41** (2): 131–139.

Mohan G, Harrison BD, Badminton RM *et al.* (1996) A confidential enquiry into deaths caused by asthma in an England health region: implications for general practice. *British Journal of General Practice* **46**: 529–532.

Ninan TK, Russell G (1992) Respiratory symptoms and atopy in Aberdeen schoolchildren: evidence from two surveys 25 years apart. *BMJ* **304**: 873–875.

Rabe KF, Vermeire PA, Soriano JB, Maier WC (2000) Clinical management of asthma in 1999: the Asthma Insights and Reality in Europe (AIRE) study. *European Respiratory Journal* **16**: 802–807.

Rambasek TE, Lang DM, Kavuru MS (2004) Omalizumab: where does it fit into current asthma management? *Cleveland Clinic Journal of Medicine* **71** (3): 251–261.

Rees J, Kanabar D (2000) ABC of Asthma. BMJ Publishing, London.

Rowe BH, Spooner C, Ducharme FM *et al*. (2001) Early emergency department treatment of acute asthma with systemic cortico-steroids (Cochrane Review). In: *The Cochrane Library Issue 3*. Oxford.

Ryan D, Freeman D (2001) *Prescribing patterns in asthmatic children in primary care*. 3M Health Care.

Storms WW (2003) Unmet needs in the treatment of allergic asthma: potential role of novel biologic therapies. *Journal of Managed Care Pharmacy* **9** (6): 534–453.

Strachan DP (2000) Family size, infection and atopy: the first decade of the hygiene hypothesis. *Thorax* **55** (Suppl. 1): S2–10.

Thole H, Kroegel C, Bassler D *et al*. (2004) The German guideline clearing project on bronchial asthma – Part 2: recommendations and key topics for a national guideline on bronchial asthma. *Pneumologie* **58** (3): 165–175.

Wareham NJ, Harrison BD, Jenkins PF *et al*. (1993) A district confidential enquiry into deaths due to asthma. *Thorax* **48**: 1117–1120.

Watanabe T, Ohta M, Murata M *et al*. (1998) Decrease in emergency room or urgent care visits due to the management of bronchial asthma inpatients and outpatients with pharmaceutical services. *Journal of Clinical Pharmacology and Therapy* **23**: 303–309.

Woodruff PG, Emond SD, Singh AK *et al*. (1998) Sudden onset severe acute asthma: clinical features and response to therapy. *Academy of Emergency Medicine* **5**: 695–701.

Chronic Obstructive Pulmonary Disease (COPD)

3

EPIDEMIOLOGY AND ECONOMIC IMPACT OF COPD

Chronic obstructive pulmonary disease (COPD) is estimated to be the fourth leading cause of death in the world (Lopez & Murray 1998), with clinical histories of the patients showing an associated and concurrent high morbidity (Barnes 2000). In the UK COPD has become a large burden on both secondary and primary health care (BTS 1997). It is a major cause of morbidity affecting an estimated 900 000 patients (NICE 2004) and causing approximately 30 000 deaths a year (ONS 2000).

The high prevalence of COPD imposes a large cost on the health service, where the direct and indirect annual costs of COPD is estimated to be £982 000 000. A further analysis of that figure indicated that the average cost per patient per annum is £819.42, with over half of this cost as a direct consequence of hospital 'inpatient' admission (NICE 2004).

The 'economic impact' is not restricted to the NHS: there are also further financial costs that have to be borne by the welfare state and the private purses of the families. It was reported that 21.9 million working days were lost in 1994–95 due to COPD (NICE 2004). In 2003 a random survey of those with COPD provided the following information: 44% of the sample were below retirement age and 24% of that cohort were completely prevented from working by COPD (Britton 2003).

The high economic and social cost is sufficient motivation to provide the driving force needed for health care professionals to seek, find and use the most efficient methods to deliver high quality care to those patients. Early diagnosis and continual effective follow-up care will not only improve the medical care given but will help to mitigate many of the medical, economic and social consequences of COPD.

This disease has also been known as chronic obstructive airway disease (COAD) or as chronic obstructive lung disease (COLD). General consensus has been reached between the UK, Europe and USA that the current title 'chronic obstructive pulmonary disease (COPD)' should be adopted (BTS 1997, GOLD Guidelines 2000, NICE 2004). The title 'chronic obstructive pulmonary disease' acknowledges that this disease does not just affect the respiratory airways; it also affects the lung parenchyma and the pulmonary circulation.

By following the more precise definition of COPD given by the new guidelines, clinicians should be able to avoid the previous practice of using COPD as a 'generic' term that could be applied to all those respiratory diseases in which the flow of air into the lungs is permanently restricted by the reduction in size or narrowing of the respiratory airways (bronchi and bronchioles). While there is considerable overlap between COPD and other respiratory diseases, such as chronic bronchitis, emphysema, and chronic asthma, each of these conditions is a disease in its own right. It is entirely possible that a patient may have one of these respiratory diseases but it may never progress further to develop into COPD (Fig. 3.1).

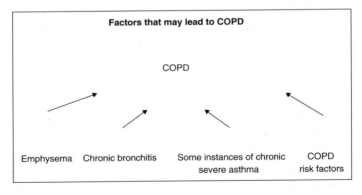

Fig. 3.1 Factors leading to COPD.

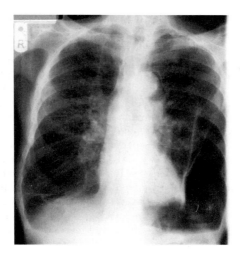

Fig. 3.2 Chest X-ray illustrating bullae.

Emphysema is a progressive destruction of alveolar septa and capillaries leading to the development of: enlarged airways and air spaces (bullae); decreased lung elastic recoil; and increased airway collapsibility. Bullae can be readily identified upon CT scan of the thorax and in some cases are visible upon chest X-ray (see Fig. 3.2).

The decrease in the ability of the lungs to recoil upon expiration often results in the airways collapsing before there can be a complete expiration of the air within the lung. Lung over-expansion then occurs when the air, trapped in air spaces that are distal to the collapsed airways, can no longer be easily expelled. It is possible to have emphysema without having COPD. However in many individuals with emphysema airway obstruction is clearly demonstrated and this then satisfies the criteria required for the diagnosis of COPD (Selby 2002).

The increase in airway obstruction observed during chronic bronchitis can be attributed to mucus hypersecretion and increased airway resistance. To aid diagnosis, a symptom approach is used. Symptoms include a cough and excessive mucus hypersecretion on most days for three successive months over two or more consecutive years (MRC 1965). Many smokers fall into this category since tobacco smoke causes irritation to airways and thus an increase in mucus production. Once airway obstruction that is not reversible is demonstrated, then a diagnosis of COPD can be considered. However a caveat has to be applied to such a diagnosis of COPD since in a proportion of those smokers who cease smoking, the airway obstruction may appear to be completely resolved and the symptoms eradicated. Not all those who smoke tobacco will develop COPD; however many will have chronic bronchitis.

Other inhaled irritants can result in a chronic productive cough. The condition used to be so common in miners subjected to continual exposure to coal mine dust, that a fit of coughing would almost pass unnoticed by others who were present. London's great smogs of the mid decades of the twentieth century caused a sudden increase in the number deaths due to respiratory illness in young and old, male or female and resulted in an overwhelming number of respiratory cases requiring admissions to London's hospitals. The crisis stimulated the enforcement of the 'Clean Air Act (ca 1953/4)' and the report of the Medical Research Council (1965). However despite general agreement and concern among health professionals and general public, 'air pollution' still remains a major factor in determining respiratory health of citizens in many countries.

There are many definitions of COPD that are used widely in clinical practice. All focus upon the fact that COPD is a disease of airflow obstruction that is not fully reversible and is progressive.

Table 3.1 provides a succinct range of definitions for COPD. The final definition given in Table 3.1 was the first to incorporate directly a specific causal agent for COPD. This is of primary importance for the management of COPD and will be referred to later in this chapter.

Table 3.1 Definitions of COPD.

A useful definition for COPD is provided in the GOLD (Global Initiative for Chronic Obstructive Lung Disease) Guidelines (2001):

'A disease state characterised by airflow limitation that is not fully reversible. The airflow limitation is usually both progressive and associated with an abnormal inflammatory response of the lungs to noxious particles or gases.'

Similar definitions have been agreed by the European Respiratory Society (ERS), American Thoracic Society (ATS) and British Thoracic Society (BTS):

'A disorder characterised by reduced maximum expiratory flow and slow forced emptying of the lungs: features that do not change markedly over several months. Most of the airflow limitation is slowly progressive and irreversible' (ERS 1995).

'A disease state characterised by the presence of airflow obstruction due to chronic bronchitis or emphysema; the airflow obstruction is generally progressive, may be accompanied by airway hyperreactivity and may be partially reversible' (ATS 1995).

'A chronic slowly progressive disorder characterised by airflow obstruction (reduced FEV_1 and FEV_1/VC ratio) that does not change markedly over several months. Most of the lung function impairment is fixed, although some reversibility can be produced by bronchodilator (or other) therapy' (BTS 1997).

'Chronic obstructive pulmonary disease (COPD) is characterised by airflow obstruction. The airflow obstruction is usually progressive, not fully reversible and does not change markedly over several months. Smoking predominantly causes the disease' (NICE 2004).

The high prevalence of COPD has encouraged a review of the British COPD guidelines culminating in the publication of the March 2004 BTS guidelines endorsed by the National Institute for Clinical Excellence (NICE). The guidelines set a precedent for the management of COPD in both primary and secondary care. This chapter incorporates many of the key points that would underpin any protocol developed from the code of clinical practice set down within the 2004 COPD guidelines.

COPD has some common features with asthma: it is a chronic disease that results in inflammatory changes in the airways. However, the airway restriction that occurs in COPD is not fully reversible (as is often the case in asthma) and of particular diagnostic and clinical importance is that COPD is a disease that is characteristically progressive, i.e. the symptoms will always become more acute with the passage of time.

Distinguishing between the progressive adverse changes that may be recognised during the clinic history of asthma and those definitive non-reversible progressive changes characteristic of COPD may be difficult. This difficulty may provide a diagnostic challenge to the health professional, but is an essential distinction to get right for the patient. It has to be made correctly to ensure that the appropriate health care is provided.

A typical example of such diagnostic difficulties may be the problem presented by a patient who has had asthma for some time, but is now failing to respond as well to asthma treatment as in the past.

The above paragraph defines the first problem that often occurs for patients with COPD. Essentially it is the practitioners' reticence to committing themselves initially to confirming the diagnosis of COPD and then initiating the correct and appropriate treatment. As with a number of chronic illnesses, often the patient may have experienced quite severe symptoms and a limitation in their activities of daily living before they seek medical advice (NICE 2004). They may well have 'accommodated' to a gradual decline in their lifestyle and not sought medical advice until a significant chest infection has dramatically reduced their ability to carry out everyday tasks.

During the consultation the patient should be asked about morning coughs; reduced exercise tolerance over a period of time; and smoking history. However, if these key questions are not explored then the patient may well not mention these symptoms. It is known that smokers seek to evade and avoid direct questions as to how many cigarettes they smoke. Consideration could then be given to whether further evidence should be gathered to investigate a possible diagnosis of COPD.

To raise the profile of COPD and prompt patients to mention early symptoms a poster has been designed by the British Lung Foundation and sent to all GP surgeries in the UK. This poster asks a few key questions which if answered 'yes' should encourage the patient to raise the matter with their GP (Fig. 3.3).

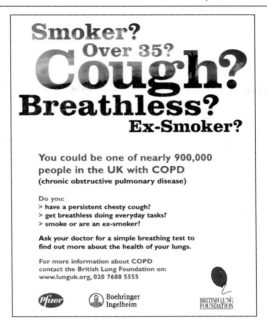

Fig. 3.3 BLF poster. With permission British Lung Foundation.

Case study: Mrs Smith, Part 1

An example of symptoms that people with COPD will tolerate prior to seeking medical intervention

Mrs Smith (aged 62) had always been a very active person. Her job, which she loved, required physical endurance and her passion of walking miles daily with her dogs ensured that she undertook vigorous daily exercise. At the age of 55 she noticed that she could not walk her dogs as far as usual before becoming exhausted, and ascribed this to the natural ageing process. At around this time she also began to wake

Continued

up each morning with a cough, which took quite a while to resolve itself after waking. Thinking that this was the expected 'smoker's cough' she did not worry unduly. She adapted by curtailing her then active lifestyle to ensure that it did not exceed her physical abilities.

A few years later her cough became more problematic and she sought the advice of her GP. Probably because of her habit of understating, the true impact of her symptoms was not discussed and salbutamol inhaler was prescribed for the symptomatic relief of her coughing.

Points for discussion

Mrs Smith was given treatment for symptomatic relief without any overt attempt to obtain any further information needed to arrive at a diagnosis. It may be that at the time of presentation Mrs Smith had either developed late onset asthma or was displaying the early symptoms of COPD. At this point these diseases can appear to display similar symptoms and it may have been difficult to provide a differential diagnosis. However the index of suspicion would suggest that, due to the smoking history of Mrs Smith, the favoured diagnosis would have been 'early COPD'. The failure to confirm a diagnosis before continuing the treatment may well have resulted in the delayed commencement of appropriate treatment.

The rate of progression of COPD can be reduced if smoking cessation advice is received early and acted upon (NICE 2004) and appropriate pulmonary rehabilitation introduced. However in this case the delay in treatment will now result in a significant long-term cost to both the NHS and to Mrs Smith, since COPD was allowed to continue unchecked. It has followed its natural rate of progress from mild to severe.

DIFFERENTIATING BETWEEN COPD AND OTHER RESPIRATORY DISEASES

As mentioned earlier, in order to diagnose COPD it is crucial that the health professional actively considers this as a possible diagnostic outcome. There will be a significantly increased chance of consideration of a COPD diagnosis if the common presenting features of the illness are determined and evaluated critically against whatever risk factors are found to be present (Halpin 2001).

Clinical history

A detailed clinical and family history should always be taken when considering a diagnosis of COPD. Consideration should be particularly paid to the existence and degree of exposure to risk factors.

Risk factors

Age

COPD rarely starts causing clinically recognisable symptoms before the age of 40. Those cases forming the rare exceptions to that generalisation are often associated with a trait that is linked to an inherited deficiency of alpha-1 antitrypsin. This disability can result in individuals developing emphysema and COPD in their twenties, that risk being enhanced if they smoke.

Smoking

This is the most common cause of COPD, and accounts for 80% of all presentations of the disease. It is thought that about 20% of people who smoke will develop COPD (Doll 1994), with the personal risk increasing with the increasing number of cigarettes smoked. With respect to smoking the amount that an individual smokes is measured in terms of 'pack years.'

A pack year = smoking 20 cigarettes per day for one year

Thus individuals who smokes 40 cigarettes a day for 1 year or those who smoked 20 cigarettes for 2 years will have accumulated the equivalent of 2 pack years.

Table 3.2 Symptoms associated with COPD.

Cough	
Breathlessness	
Chest tightness	} Limited variability
Wheeze	
Sputum production	

Genetic and family background
Weak family links have been established (Bellamy 2003, Silverman 2001), unlike those found in asthma in which a prior history of asthma in the family is regarded an important risk factor.

Patients often have a range of symptoms. However the most common that are associated with COPD are listed in Table 3.2.

In COPD these symptoms are characteristically insidious during onset, occurring over a period of months; they are fairly stable and persistent, slowly progressive and never return to normal and become worse with exertion.

CLINICAL EXAMINATION
Chest auscultation may reveal generalised widespread wheeze, with perhaps a hyperinflated chest. However chest examination may be completely normal in cases of mild COPD. Severe COPD may provide clinical symptoms on examination of peripheral oedema, central cyanosis, use of accessory muscles to breath, cachexia, weight loss, wheeze or quiet breath sounds and increased respiratory rate. Finger clubbing may be present in some cases.

In the past patients with COPO have been thought of as either blue bloaters or pink puffers. Those 'descriptive classifications' should be seen as the extreme manifestations of COPD with most patients existing between those two ends of the spectrum. *Pink puffers* are those patients who 'strive' to maintain relatively normal blood gases by breathing hard and fast. This is often quite distressing to both the patient and those who observe this respiratory response. *Blue bloaters* are patients with COPD who are 'acclimatised' to their abnormal blood gases and physiologically accept hypoxaemia and hypercapnia by the reduction in their regulatory centre's 'desire' to breath. The position between these two types of physiological response occupied by the patient is not under the conscious control of the patient. However exercising their choice in continuing some of the activities they consider enhance their quality of life, such as continuing to smoke, may play some part in determining their position on that spectrum. Associated with blue bloaters are the related systemic effects of COPD such as pulmonary hypertension, peripheral oedema and cor pulmonale (Ward *et al.* 2002).

Objective tests to be used in aiding the diagnosis of COPD

Lung function tests

It is diagnostically important to be able to demonstrate that airflow limitation is present in the case of COPD. This is usually done using both spirometry and peak expiratory flow rate (PEF). Some debate exists as to the merit of using PEF as a clinical guide in COPD patients, with the 2004 NICE guidelines advocating the sole use of spirometry as a measurement of COPD disease progression. Within primary care a number of GPs advocate the routine use of PEF (to monitor COPD disease progression, arguing it is a more reliable and accurate test in primary care (Chavannes 2004). However the result of the development of portable digital spirometers together with improved access to training will ensure the greater use of spirometry in primary care.

Peak expiratory flow rate is usually measured by a peak flow meter. In some cases when COPD is suspected it is worth considering using a paediatric peak flow meter. This is beneficial when recording smaller volume outputs by providing an appropriate scale for greater accuracy. This is particularly useful where initially an adult peak flow meter records low inconsistent readings or there are difficulties in getting the patient to form a tight seal around the mouthpiece of the adult peak flow meter.

It is important to note that whereas a normal value of peak expiratory flow rate on its own does not exclude a diagnosis of COPD, a normal FEV_1 measured via spirometry will exclude a diagnosis of COPD.

Spirometry

NICE (2004) advocate the use of spirometry as being essential to diagnose and assess the severity of COPD. Table 3.3 includes definitions of the fundamental lung functions that may be quantified by the use of spirometry. The key results obtained from spirometry that would support a diagnosis of COPD are:

FEV_1 of less than 80% of predicted value;
and a FEV_1/FVC ratio of less than 70%.

Please refer to Fig. 3.4 for examples of spirometry data indicating either the absence or presence of airflow obstruction.

The GOLD guidelines categorically state, unless the patient fulfils the criteria indicating airflow obstruction then they do not have COPD. However, the GOLD guidelines have introduced the 'at risk' group of COPD patients to flag those patients who have at that point normal spirometry readings but whose clinical records show some of the diagnostic persistent symptoms listed in Table 3.2.

Figure 3.4 provides a schema for spirometry volume–time curves indicating normal airflow and the typical results obtained where there is mild or severe airflow obstruction. There is no fundamental difference between the volume-time curves obtained between those plotted when airflow obstruction is the result of asthma or the consequence of COPD.

Spirometry is however a powerful quantitative tool when 'reversibility testing' is used to confirm the correct diagnosis. The distinction can be made by comparing the results of spirometry obtained during the episode of respiratory debility with those obtained after there has been some period of recovery. In the case of asthma the 'reversibility testing' will show that an improvement has occurred following recovery; the numerical data obtained may lie within the normal upper and lower

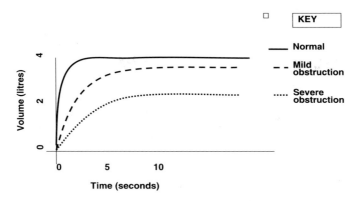

Fig. 3.4 Spirometry indicating airflow obstruction.

Table 3.3 Spirometric measurements of lung function.

FEV_1: forced expired volume in the first second of expiration.
FVC: forced vital capacity is the total volume of air that can be expired.
FEV_1/FVC ratio:
   (FEV_1%): the % of FVC expelled in the first second of expiration (normally around 80%).
FEV_1% predicted:
   value individualised to the patient which compares his or her.
   FEV_1 with the predicted value for a person of their age, height and gender.

With permission from *Airways Journal* (Bellamy 2003).

bounds. This would not be typical of COPD where the data will indicate little improvement has occurred.

MANAGEMENT GOALS FOR THOSE WITH COPD

The primary therapeutic goals for patients with COPD are reducing symptoms, increasing function and improving the quality of life (Halpin 2001, NICE 2004). This is based on the concept, as discussed previously, that COPD is a progressive incurable disease with little demonstrable modification of its

Table 3.4 Differential diagnosis of asthma and COPD.

	ASTHMA	COPD
Age at onset	Any	Mainly above 40 years old
Smoking history	✓ ×	✓✓
Family history of atopy/asthma	✓✓	✓ ×
Presence of hayfever and eczema	✓✓	✓ ×
Intermittent symptoms from trigger factors	✓✓	× ×
Nocturnal symptoms	✓✓	✓ ×
Symptoms constant	× ×	✓✓
Symptoms progressive	✓ ×	✓✓
PEF variable	✓✓	✓ ×
Responsive to bronchodilator	✓✓	✓ ×
Responsive to corticosteroid	✓✓	✓ ×

Key

✓✓ = high probability of factors present.

✓ × = factors may or may not be present.

× × = factors not present.

Redrawn with permission from Bellamy D (2003) How to differentiate asthma from COPD in primary care. *Airways Journal* **1:** 10–14.

course by the use of modern therapy. Thus having made the diagnosis of COPD the health professional has to be able to address the issues that abound in the support and management of the patient with COPD.

Assessment of the impact of COPD to patients

A holistic approach

COPD is a life-limiting disease. As already discussed it has a significant impact upon morbidity and mortality of those who have the disease. Patients who have the disease should receive holistic support from the health care professionals that they encounter.

It is important to note that COPD is not a curable disease. The goal of treatment is to minimise the progression of the disease, reduce the presence of symptoms and maximise physical function and quality of life. This has immediate psychological effect upon the individual with COPD who may, up to the diagnosis of this disease, have had all their health problems completely resolved following their consultation with the appropriate health professionals (Nicassio & Smith 1995, Kleme Leidy *et al.* 1990).

All patients who have COPD will have their own unique health needs; however there are a number of common issues that should be addressed by health professionals. These should focus upon reducing symptoms; maintaining or improving quality of life; nutritional support and dietary advice; supplying health advice and clear information for the patient concerning the use of medication; disease progression; the stratagems and support available to aid smoking cessation; and the ways of buffering the impact that the illness is having upon their life and their family (NICE 2004, BTS 1997, GOLD 2001).

Primary care is often the patient's first port of call, seeking the advice of their practice nurse, GP or other health professional. Since the primary care is the arena in which most of the care for COPD occurs, these health professionals have a key and fundamental role to play in the management of COPD. This relationship will in most cases be the mainstay of health care for the patient with COPD. Since primary care team is effectively the only conduit that can lead to the correct, rapid and appropriate diagnosis of COPD, then investigations, using the criteria and methodology discussed above, should be carried out in all cases in which there is any index of suspicion that the patient has COPD.

Any health professional should be able to assess the risk factors to which the COPD patient is exposed and ascertain from the patient those key issues that are causing them concern (Seamark *et al.* 2001). It may be that the patient should be referred to others working in secondary care for spirometry, chest X-ray and related advice, but once these are carried out then the initial care is often placed back within the realm of primary care. Many primary care units now have the facilities and trained practice nurses to carry out spirometry promptly, adeptly and efficiently. Usually secondary care only deals with any acute exacerbations of COPD and end-stage COPD. Tertiary care for those who require it is an important issue to be considered as part of the care package for COPD (Gibbons *et al.* 2001).

Assessment tools

Much research has been invested in an attempt to try and provide an assessment tool that will help all health professionals recognise and evaluate the health status of the patient. Health status is more than the presence or absence of symptoms; it is much more subjectively evaluated by the patients using both qualitative and quantitative criteria. It involves how much the individual has been forced to accept adaptation or compromise in the attempt to continue to actively pursue the normal activities of daily life; how bothered they are by their disease and what they consider to be an acceptable or bearable level of symptoms to tolerate before needing to return to their primary care clinic. The latter point is particular important with COPD since as the disease deteriorates it becomes increasingly difficult to alleviate all the symptoms that the patient is experiencing.

The two most important questionnaires or 'assessment tools' that are frequently employed to assess COPD are: the Chronic Respiratory Disease Questionnaire (CRQ) and the St George's Respiratory Questionnaire (SGRQ). Other COPD specific instruments exist but they measure basically the same domains as the two questionnaires given above, an indication that there is a relatively broad consensus regarding the parameters most affected by this disease.

However, these assessment tools are only aids and their merit lies in the fact that they are reproducible and can thus be replicated by any health professional without causing significant bias. There is generally a good correlation between the questionnaires and the physiological measurements from spirometry (ZuWallack 2003). They do not, however, replace or diminish the need for good appropriate assessment being made at an individual level by a health professional.

HEALTH CARE PROFESSIONAL TREATMENT ISSUES OF COPD

Tobacco smoking cessation will significantly reduce the rates of decline in lung function and in the patient's exercise tolerance. Such steep rates of decline are frequently associated with the deteriorating COPD (NICE 2004). It has been repeatedly shown that giving up smoking does reduce the rate of decline in both FEV_1 (Scanlon *et al.* 2000) and disease morbidity (Sethi *et al.* 2000). Smoking cessation advice should be offered routinely to all who smoke and in particular directed to those with COPD (West *et al.* 2000).

Primary care is best placed to provide such advice (Ashcroft 2003) and the role of the practice nurse in undertaking this task has been encouraged by both the NHS and those independent agencies such as the pharmaceutical companies that work in conjunction with the Health Service. Utilising the therapeutic relationship that the primary care team will be developing with the patient enhances the degree to which the maintenance of smoking cessation support is accepted and improved. However, since all health professionals should promote smoking cessation advice, this united front will further reinforce patient confidence in this advice (West *et al.* 2000). Opportunistic discussion between health professional and patient should not be under-rated (Percival 2004).

Patients should be directed towards other groups or sources of help if further support is found to be necessary. Quitline began as a London based organisation designed to help Londoners to stop smoking. It now provides a national free-phone service and will run health professional based smoking cessation courses, tailored to meet individual organisational needs (QUIT 2004). For further information, QUIT may be contacted directly (see address list in Appendix C).

The availability of pharmacological adjuncts such as nicotine patches and bupropion has significantly increased smoking quit rates (Halpin 2001). The National Institute for Clinical Excellence (NICE) has published guidance which advocated that both these products should become available, on NHS prescription, to those smokers that express a desire to quit (NICE 2002).

PHARMACOLGICAL MANAGEMENT OF COPD

The options

Bronchodilators are found to be of practical use in the management of COPD, although as discussed previously much of the airflow restriction is shown not to be reversible. The symptomatic relief that the patients with COPD experience is often substantial (Cook *et al.* 2001), reducing breathlessness and increasing exercise tolerance. It has been suggested that the bronchodilators may effect those changes in airflow restriction that are too small for spirometry to detect as changes in FEV_1, but still significant enough to reduce the hyperinflation associated with COPD.

Short-acting bronchodilators

Short-acting bronchodilators (β_2 agonists), such as salbutamol and terbutaline, are effective for no more than four hours by acting directly upon the smooth muscle of the bronchial airways and are usually the first-line therapy for COPD. They are either administered pro ra nate (as needed) or at regular intervals to aid in symptom management of patients requiring other therapy (Sestini *et al.* 2000).

Long-acting bronchodilators

Long-acting bronchodilators (β_2 agonists) such as salmeterol or formoterol have a similar mechanism of action to the short-acting bronchodilators mentioned above, but their effect will last for about 12 hours. In some patients they produce more profound improvements, increasing FEV_1 by 100–200 mL, and substantially improving health status and breathlessness scores (Halpin 2004). Their effects would appear to be dose-dependent and maximum improvement in health status is produced by salmeterol 50 micrograms or formoterol 12 micrograms b.d. (Dahl *et al.* 2001, Jones and Bosh 1997). These bronchodilators should be used for the management of patients who remain symptomatic on short-acting β_2 agonists. However they are more expensive than short-acting β_2 agonists and they are not at present available in a formulation that will allow nebulisation. They are not used in the treatment of acute exacerbations. Based on current practice, those patients who are using long-acting β_2 agonists are encouraged to continue to take this medication during an acute exacerbation.

Short-acting anticholinergics

These drugs cause bronchodilation by blocking the bronchoconstriction effect signalled by the cholinergic nerves within the lungs. The cholinergic tone of the lungs (of COPD patients) increases at rest and it is the reduction in this tone that produces the major bronchodilator effect in COPD patients. The clinical advantages conferred by the use of 'short-acting anticholinergic' drugs should now confirm their right to be considered to be the treatment of first choice in COPD patients. In practice they are prescribed less frequently than the short-acting β_2 agonists. Halpin (2004) suggests that this is due to the greater familiarity of practitioners in the prescription of short-acting β_2 agonists.

There are benefits to be derived when anticholinergics ipratropium bromide and oxitropium are prescribed for the regular use of patients with COPD. They were shown to be capable of producing stable sustained bronchodilation for up to eight hours. It has to be noted that the speed of onset is slower than short-acting β_2 agonists, and this may be one of the factors influencing the apparent preference of practitioners noted by Halpin. Anticholinergics are available as nebulisation therapy and are effectively used to treat exacerbations of COPD.

Long-acting anticholinergics

Tiotropium is at present the only long-acting anticholinergic bronchodilator available for prescription. It has been widely advocated and clinical trials have shown it to be effective in the management of COPD (Vincken *et al.* 2002). It reduces breathlessness and improves both exercise tolerance and health status.

Patient compliance

Generally medication that requires once or twice daily dosing improves patient compliance/concordance. The ensuring of patient concordance is often the biggest issue that has to be overcome and addressed; it is self-evident that medication that requires minimal patient concordance should become the medication of first choice. However the NICE 2004 guidelines suggest that in mild COPD the short-acting β_2 agonists should remain the medication of first choice. When moderate to severe COPD occurs or when patients remain symptomatic, especially in cases where breathless is involved, then long-acting bronchodilators should be considered for substitution into their drug regime. Assessment should be followed up regarding the management of patients' COPD no later than one month after the commencement of new medication (Halpin 2004, Donahue *et al.* 2002). Long-acting bronchodilators have been proven to reduce the frequency of acute exacerbations and associated hospital admission rates; they may thus prove to be far more cost effective in the long term.

Drug delivery systems are discussed in detail in Chapter 4; however inhaled medication via pressure metered dose canisters remains the most common method of drug delivery. Nebulisation therapy is advantages in acute exacerbation management if respiratory effort is arduous and respiratory rate is high.

Methylxanthines, such as theophylline, are used in the treatment of COPD; however their use is perhaps of limited value and they are generally reserved for the treatment of end-stage COPD.

Steroid medication

Oral steroid maintenance medication may have some benefit in a small cohort of those with stable COPD (Peperall *et al.* 1997). However, the side effects associated with long-term oral steroid therapy may outweigh the benefits confirmed. These side effects include: weight gain; osteoporosis; diabetes; hypertension; and easy bruising (Griffiths & Jordan 2002). These outcomes should be clearly explained to all patients who are about to receive this medication. Additional medication for the alleviation or reduction of these side effects, particularly that of osteoporosis, may be considered a useful adjunct.

Inhaled steroids may be of some benefit in stable COPD. Where spirometry has been used to measure the primary outcome of inhaled steroids, there has been no evidence of a proven change to the rate of decline in FEV_1 following their use. Consideration of other factors however indicate that there may be a clinical benefit to patients with severe COPD by the addition of inhaled steroids, such as a reduction in exacerbation rates (Burge *et al.* 2000). Guidelines would suggest that inhaled steroids should be reserved for those patients with severe COPD ($FEV_1 < 40\%$ predicted value) and frequent exacerbations (NICE 2004).

Management of COPD exacerbations

'An exacerbation is a sustained worsening of the patient's symptoms from his or her usual stable state that is beyond normal day to day variations, and is acute in onset. Commonly reported symptoms are worsening breathlessness, cough, increased sputum production and change in sputum colour. The change in these symptoms often necessitates a change in medication.' (NICE 2004; p. 131).

BTS guidelines

The 2004 BTS guidelines provide detailed information and guidance on the management of COPD exacerbations. Such clearly presented information will help the primary health care team to decide whether to place the patient in hospital or manage the exacerbation in the patient's home. The decision will be dependent on the severity of patient symptoms and take into account the infrastructure and support available to the patient. Many patients can be managed effectively and competently by the primary care team. It is hoped that such clearly outlined protocols and the unbiased critical review of the patient's condition will help to reduce the frequency of hospital admissions. At the time of writing there has not been any research undertaken evaluating what impact the 2004

COPD guidelines have upon the management of COPD exacerbations.

Whether treated at home or in a hospital the principal tenets of COPD exacerbation treatment are the same. These are to alleviate symptoms, treat any infection that may be present and hasten recovery. While patients remain at home they should be reviewed regularly and any deterioration in symptoms should alert the carer to consider whether those treated at home now require hospital admission.

Antibiotics

Antibiotic therapy is often prescribed for COPD exacerbations, with antibiotic choice dependent upon local policies, but generally revolving around the preferred use of amoxicillin, clarithromycin or trimethoprim (Halpin 2001). Usually a seven-day course is adequate, but those patients who have repeated infections should perhaps be given a reserve supply of antibiotic. Treatment could then be started at home immediately there was a re-appearance of symptoms. Oral steroid medication may have value in this instance, since the principles of reducing the airway inflammation present in an infected airway still remain valid in COPD.

Bronchodilators

Increased breathlessness usually can be managed either by the addition of regular short-acting bronchodilators or by increasing the frequency with which they are used. The use of nebulisers to deliver the inhaled medication is routinely used in the hospital setting; however if the patient is able to maintain a good inhaler technique by using a large volume spacer, then this method has been shown to be as effective as nebulisation therapy (Bee *et al.* 2001).

Hospital admission

Hospital admission still has the advantage of allowing further investigations to be carried out and in some instances these may provide a very positive benefit to patients by their consequential inclusion into the follow-up services. These outreach, home-care teams are the mainstay of those patients with severe COPD, and they are important for all respiratory chronic ill health management.

Hospital admissions allow the opportunity for specific follow up investigations to be carried out immediately. These can include: chest X-ray; full blood count; urea, electrolytes and arterial blood gas analyses; ECG; sputum culture; and further spirometry. The information obtained can then be interpreted de nouveau against the backdrop of the drug regimen, the symptoms displayed and the exacerbation progression.

Further benefits accrue from the hospital setting where monitored oxygen therapy can be given more easily, safely and rapidly than it could be delivered at home. In hospital such oxygen therapy could be given concomitantly with the administration of the medication via nebulisation. Oxygen therapy should be used advisedly and should achieve a PaO_2 of at least 6.6 kPa, without significant rise in the $PaCO_2$. Until arterial gas tensions are known, oxygen therapy should be given at a percentage concentration of 24–28% via a Venturi mask. Once arterial blood gas tensions are available then the percentage of inspired oxygen administered should be adjusted accordingly. Chapter 5 discusses in more detail oxygen delivery systems and the principles of oxygen therapy.

If respiratory failure develops then non-invasive ventilatory support (NIV) should be considered. These include continuous positive airway pressure (CPAP) and bi-phasic airway pressure (BiPAP). Non-invasive ventilatory support is usually delivered via a mask that covers the nose, but may be delivered via a mask that covers both the nose and the mouth. Research indicates that for those patients with acute severe exacerbation of COPD, the NIV support decreases mortality; reduces the need for intubation; shows improvement of pH; results in fewer complications and a shorter duration of stay in hospital (Ram *et al.* 2003).

However if facilities for these non-invasive support measures are not available then intubation should be considered against the backdrop of co-morbidities, patient exacerbation history and health status. When full intubation and related systemic support are considered it should be fully discussed with the patient and their family before the commencement of the procedures, with clear ceilings agreed to the level of treatment to be given to the patient (NICE 2004). This allows for the patient and family to discuss their wishes and be involved in the treatment decision options (BTS 2002).

Unfortunately once a patient has experienced one exacerbation of their COPD they are likely to experience others; more than three a year will have a significant effect upon the rates of FEV_1 decline and COPD disease progression (Donaldson *et al.* 2002).

DISCHARGE PLANNING

Early discussions with the patient and family on what they could contribute towards the establishment of a planned supportive discharge will reduce the probability of the patient becoming re-admitted due to an inability to cope at home with their current COPD exacerbation (Sin & Tu 2000, Lau *et al.* 2001). By establishing a liaison with the whole health professional team and receiving an introduction to the effective utilisation of pulmonary rehabilitation programmes, hospital at home schemes, assisted discharge facilities and respiratory outreach teams, the ability of patients and families to cope at home will improve (Gravil *et al.* 1998, Hermiz *et al.* 2002). Often the use of such services encourages the development not only of self-management strategies, but also strengthens their confidence in their own ability to recognise adverse events regarding their COPD and sharpens their recognition of the need to seek appropriate medical advice early.

Written and verbal advice should be made available to the patient and their families, and several charities produce excellent booklets/leaflets that are freely available. For example the British Lung Foundation produce a succinct 16-page booklet entitled 'Living with COPD' that addresses many issues that health professionals overlook when discussing COPD with patients, such as the importance of wearing suitable unrestrictive clothing, or sitting down when getting dressed.

NUTRITIONAL STATUS

Body mass index

It is important to highlight nutritional status when considering the holistic management of patients with COPD. Research has indicated that many people with severe COPD have a significant and progressive weight loss, as defined by a weight loss of 5–10% over a year (Hugh & Fitting 2003). Between 27% (Braun *et al.* 1984) and 47% (Hunter *et al.* 1981) of patients have a weight loss of this magnitude.

Nutritional status is routinely measured in clinical situations by a consideration of Body Mass Index (BMI) which is the numerical ratio of body weight (kg) divided by height (m) squared:

$$BMI = \frac{Weight\,(kg)}{Height\,(m)^2}$$

Nutritional depletion is often considered to have occurred when the BMI is less than $18\,kg\,m^{-2}$ (Jones *et al.* 1988). Several of the changes in the physiological processes that characterise COPD have been suggested as the possible causal agents responsible for the loss in weight in these patients. Thus the laboured breathing that is associated with COPD indicates not only the greater use of accessory muscles, but also an increase in the rate and depth of breathing. These changes have been cited as a possible reason for an extra energy expenditure needed to fuel such an increased workload. However while it is accepted that the above respiratory behaviour could have an effect, it is uncertain that while the patient is at rest, their increased extra energy expenditure could reach values as high as those often suggested. Such changes in physiological response may not be the only or major cause of resting hypermetabolism.

Metabolic rate

The medication used to treat COPD may be responsible for an increased resting metabolic rate. It has been shown that β_2 agonists increase resting metabolic rate; however tolerance to these effects is usually reached in eight weeks. Theophylline has been shown to increase resting metabolic rate in healthy subjects but no evidence has been obtained to indicate a corresponding increase occurs in those patients with COPD (Mosier *et al.* 1996).

It is likely that the weight loss experienced by those patients with severe COPD will be shown to have multifactorial causes. The weight loss does not limit itself to a reduction in body fat composition; it is more widespread and has a significant effect upon the composition of skeletal and respiratory muscle composition (Lansen 2003), lung parenchyma and fat regulation (Schiffelers & Blaak 2003). Thus while the consequential reduction in functional skeletal and respiratory muscle may be a significant factor in limiting the exercise capacity of those with COPD, the presence of abnormal lung parenchyma may well be responsible for a significant part of the increase in the chronicity of COPD.

It has been suggested that the role of leptin is crucial in the management and regulation of nutritional status and metabolic rate in normal subjects, and it is reasonable to conclude that it is no less so in those patients with COPD. Leptin is a protein synthesised by adipose tissue and it has been postulated that its role is to provide the signal to the hypothalamus that results in increased energy expenditure, glucose metabolism, and increased fat metabolism (Creutzberg 2003). Leptin is known to be an 'energy balance' regulating hormone (Campfield *et al.* 1996). Further research into the role that leptin plays in maintaining the nutritional status in patients with COPD seems to be indicated.

Increased mortality

Regardless of the apparent degree of disease severity, clinical studies and population studies have indicated that the involuntary weight loss and being underweight are correlated to increased mortality (Schols *et al.* 1998). In order to avoid the progression of functional decline among COPD patients, it is important to optimise the treatment of those patients who are underweight by detecting and reversing the weight loss as soon as possible, and then implementing effective longer term measures to avoid any further loss of weight (Smit *et al.* 1999).

This later stratagem may be effected by introducing several interlocking and interdependent measures that may be summarised thus: increasing dietary intake and/or by altering dietary habits to include different (energy-dense) foods; and finding the optimum practical timing of meals or snacks in relation to the individual patient's symptoms, to ensure they are provided at the periods when appetite is at its optimum. The Mediterranean diet, particularly the consumption of wholegrains, fruits and vegetables has been shown to moderate the progression of COPD (Collins 2003). However acceptance of an alteration of diet relies upon effecting a change in the health beliefs of patients and possibly consequential changes in their social behaviour, since the choice of diet and the protocols of dining remains an important and essential component of social behaviour for many people.

Dietary advice

There may be powerful hidden agendas that have to be addressed in relation to the initial weight loss experienced by those with COPD, since this may be met with positive feedback from peers and family as it may be seen by them as desirable and socially advantageous to be slim. The patients themselves might have earlier expressed their intention of trying to lose weight, possibly believing that this would alleviate or reduce their symptoms. Those patients with weight loss will have to be persuaded to adopt an eating pattern outside the social norm, by accepting the need for a regular intake of high-energy foods (Schols 2003).

However, the greatest effect of this changed attitude to diet may be noticed in the increased emphasis being placed upon the earlier detection of patients with COPD and importance of giving dietary advice at that point. This change would occur simultaneously at all levels of patient care, be it at home, in outpatients clinics, or in primary care and acute secondary care settings. All health professionals should be able to liaise together to provide dietary advice appropriate to those patients with COPD (Collins 2003). All these objectives should be placed high on the agenda of goals agreed among the health professionals whose specialised roles would then interlock and work in unity, doing much to ensure that a higher success rate could be achieved by gaining patient co-operation and dietary self-management. Effecting such an attitude change, goal setting and establishing a working feedback system would do much to prevent patient relapses (Schols & Burg 2003).

PULMONARY REHABILITATION

'Pulmonary rehabilitation can be defined as a multi-disciplinary programme of care for patients with chronic respiratory impairment that is individually tailored and designed to optimise each patient's physical and social performance and autonomy'(NICE 2004, p. 84).

Pulmonary rehabilitation leads to improvements in: health related quality of life; functional exercise capacity and maximum exercise capacity (Lacasse *et al.* 1997). Within the UK, pulmonary rehabilitation programmes were initially established in secondary care settings. However after the emergence of Primary Care Trusts (PCTs), pulmonary rehabilitation programmes became increasingly more available in the primary care arena (Donner & Decramer 2003). The major issues that are discussed and actively addressed within such pulmonary rehabilitation programmes include smoking cessation, measurement of functional health status and methods of securing its improvement. Associated topics and programmes are developed in ways that are found to be most appropriate to each individual patient. Such programmes generally review and act upon the latest information and recommendations on the management of: medication therapy; nutrition; training of peripheral muscle to aid in maintaining mobility and help with the work of breathing; exercise training per se; physiotherapy; educational and psychological support. It is thus self-evident that this approach requires a dedicated multiprofessional team resolved and able not only to encourage open, frank and good communication between all the health professionals involved, but also to be equally responsive and sensitive to the comments, questions and fears of the patients and their families.

Pulmonary rehabilitation is not primarily a programme for the establishment of forums or focus groups, although this may be considered to be a consequential advantage that may help to attain its principal objectives. Each programme of direct and active intervention is designed by a team consisting of specialised care professionals, the patient and the carers for use with a specific individual. The main objective is to use the individual skills present in the teams so that they are co-ordinated and mutually supportive in their efforts to obtain the optimum quality of life possible for patients with COPD.

The NICE 2004 guidelines suggest that pulmonary rehabilitation programmes should be made available for all appropriate patients, and to all those that consider themselves disabled by COPD. However it is not suitable for those who are unable to walk, or have co-morbidities of severe cardiac disease.

Nurse specialists and respiratory physiotherapists have a crucial role to play in ensuring that pulmonary rehabilitation programmes are initiated within health care settings, that the recruited patients attend as required, and that they have a programme of rehabilitation prescribed to suit their needs.

Early supported discharge and hospital at home services often naturally link into such pulmonary rehabilitation programmes and provide the mainstay of COPD care in the primary care setting. Nurse-led services have been demonstrated to significantly decrease the rate of hospital readmission (Gibbons *et al.* 2001) and improve patient quality of life (Gibbons & Bartley 2003).

SEVERE/END-STAGE COPD

Palliative care

The progressive nature of COPD will often lead to a debilitating and severe end-stage of life. At this stage palliative care options should be addressed. Health care professionals should consider: reducing symptoms; pain relief; anxiety; coping strategies and breathing retraining and relaxation therapies. Long-term oxygen therapy (LTOT) should be provided to allow the patient to have a degree of function at home and carry out some of their activities of daily living. Chapter 5 considers the principles of LTOT therapy in more detail.

Palliative care will provide support for both the patient and the family and its value should not be understated. However the provision of palliative care is limited at present in the case of end-stage COPD. The good practice and example set by palliative care in instances of lung cancer should be emulated, and become freely available for all end-stage respiratory disease.

Case study: Mrs Smith, Part 2

Several years after her first consultation with her GP, Mrs Smith had her first exacerbation of what subsequently was confirmed as COPD. It was only following upon that exacerbation that a firm clinical diagnosis of COPD was ascribed to her. Despite symptoms of chronic persistent productive cough, reduced exercise tolerance and the use of all accessory muscles to breath whilst carrying out the routine tasks of living, the early diagnosis was not confirmed.

Mrs Smith had continued in her active job, but had resigned herself to not undertaking any of the household chores and merely existing in the home environment. Mrs Smith's only medication up to this point had remained salbutamol for symptomatic relief.

Mrs Smith's exacerbation resulted in her being unable to talk without difficulty, walk or mobilise and then she collapsed at home, requesting an emergency call be made for an ambulance. Upon arrival the ambulance crew found a severely clinically distressed individual; they immediately commenced oxygen therapy since pulse oximetry and clinical observation clearly revealed a significant degree of cyanosis (peripheral pulse oximetry of 82%). Mrs Smith was taken to the primary care-based local hospital and not to the further away secondary care hospital. The reasons for this are many, but focus upon the patient's wishes and the clinical need for rapid assessment by a qualified medical physician. Mrs Smith was seen and prescribed nebulised

---

salbutamol, ipratropium bromide and maintenance oxygen therapy. After several successive nebulisations Mrs Smith improved, but remained adamant that she did not want to be transferred for further treatment in a secondary care setting. The physician expressed his wish that she remained in hospital but conceded to the choice expressed by his health professional patient that she wished her treatment to be continued at home. The family were given strict instructions that should they feel concerned or if there was any deterioration in Mrs Smith's condition at home they should phone for an ambulance immediately and not wait to phone the doctor or hospital for further confirmation.

The GP organised a home nebuliser for Mrs Smith and appropriate medication, but no-one ensured that Mrs Smith's family were told how this equipment operated. Mrs Smith was given oral antibiotic therapy for her productive cough.

Review was undertaken every third day by the GP, who had been assured by Mrs Smith that she would be able to travel to the practice. Mrs Smith returned from the primary care-based hospital and went to bed exhausted, her breathing laboured and unable to talk.

Her recovery from this her first exacerbation was long and arduous. It took two months from the onset of the exacerbation before she could return to her work, and four months later she still experienced significant reduction in the range of activity that she had enjoyed prior to her exacerbation. There was no follow-up after the initial exacerbation, no suggestion of pulmonary rehabilitation and limited review of current medication.

Points for discussion/consideration

- What effect has the inappropriate treatment for Mrs Smith's COPD symptoms had upon her disease progression?
- Was primary care the best place for Mrs Smith's care in respect to her exacerbation?

Continued

- Prescribing medication is of limited use if no-one demonstrates how to use the equipment. Should one presume that no prior knowledge exists?
- Would COPD information on pulmonary rehabilitation, disease progression and the current medication guidelines be sufficient to inform and aid in the duty of care entrusted to the primary care centre?
- Is Mrs Smith likely to have another exacerbation of COPD, which could have been prevented or reduced had the 2004 NICE guidelines been followed?

THE PATIENT'S EXPERIENCE OF COPD

It is important in considering any chronic ill health disease that the needs and wishes of the patient are addressed. Indeed the 'Expert Patient' document (DOH 2001) places patients paramount with regard to becoming the expert in their disease, and they are of course the fountainhead of all knowledge in respect of their own current concerns. Common themes/issues that patients want to address are given in Table 3.5. These are wide-ranging, are of utmost importance to the individuals concerned, and illustrate the more common issues raised by those with COPD.

Table 3.5 Some aims of patients with COPD.

Get off oxygen.
Keep healthy.
Do the things I want to do.
Do my gardening.
Play with my grandchildren.
Breathe better.
Walk without getting short of breath.
Go to my daughter's wedding.
Not have to carry oxygen around in the car.
Dance with my wife.
Have a conversation without having to stop and gasp for breath.
Not be so tired all the time.

Health beliefs

Chronic illness will challenge the individual's health beliefs (Cooper 2001). Since COPD cannot be 'escaped' this challenge will be made daily and continue throughout the lifetime of the patient. The aim of any treatment is directed towards to the relieving of symptoms; initially this is often achieved quite successfully, thereby frequently promoting a sense of wellbeing. However the challenge returns when, as the disease progresses, the treatment that has previously been working well now appears to be failing to relieve those symptoms.

Health beliefs of the individual should be explored and discussed with the patient. It is important to note that in any initial conversations with the individual, confronting what the health professional perceives to be an inappropriate health belief of the patient may not necessarily be appropriate and may even be counterproductive. Health promotion and empowerment suggest that the patient should have their health beliefs respected, but be given the appropriate information that allows them to develop their own coping strategies for the disease. The health professional may have ready access within the Health Authority to well-established networks for the support of patients with COPD and chronic ill health. It would be advantageous for the primary health carers to be aware of this type of support, and to be able to facilitate its uptake and its acceptance by their patients. Nationally there are organisations that exist for advice such as the British Lung Foundation, Action on Smoking and Health (ASH) and QUIT who provide smoking cessation advice.

Support network

As health professionals we only see the patient continually for those brief periods when their disease is bothersome, and when treatment and active intervention is required. The patient however has to cope with COPD continuously for 24 hours a day, seven days a week. If the patient has the advantage of a good social support network they are likely to cope better with this disease and have less hospital admissions than other patients who do not have such home support (Holman & Lorig

2000). Support does not necessarily come from family members alone but can be given by neighbours, friends and colleagues. An accurate evaluation of the resources such carers can contribute in terms of its quantity, quality, strengths and expertise should be part of any nursing care assessment carried out.

SELF-MANAGEMENT OF COPD

Table 3.6 highlights some of the important topics that the health professional and the patient with COPD must discuss and explore before suggesting any practical stratagems that will enable the patient and family to effectively cope with COPD at home and in their daily life.

As COPD progresses it may begin to exert a very real debilitating physical and psychological effect on the patient. They may have to give up participating in tasks that they have felt are the very essence of their wellbeing. The forced adaptations that have to be made will continue to intrude relentlessly into their work, hobbies and partnership. To aid their mobility, a cascade of changes may be necessary: they may have to move their home; have mobility aids placed in their houses; have home oxygen installed; and agree to the need to modify their

Table 3.6 Self-management tasks of patients with COPD.

Recognising/responding to symptoms
Monitoring physical indicators
Controlling triggers to symptoms
Using medication
Managing acute episodes
Maintaining nutrition and diet
Maintaining adequate exercise/activity
Giving up smoking
Using less stressful techniques
Seeking information
Adapting to work
Managing relationships with significant others
Managing emotions and psychological responses

From Clark *et al.* (1991).

car. As the disease progresses patients may cease driving, becoming house bound due to the fatigue and extreme breathlessness experienced after any kind of exertion.

House moving for example is a major challenge for the fit and becomes even more so when coping with chronic ill health. The practical advantages that may seem to be gained by moving, must not be allowed to become outweighed by the losses of any of the underpinning social advantages on which the individuals have depended to sustain their quality of life. Each forced change has an impact on the patient's self-esteem and ability to cope. Any assessment must recognise the degree of social support and friendships that are present and utilised as key social support for those with COPD. The decision to move must consider the myriad of issues both for and against such a decision and the wishes of the patient and their family.

ALTERNATIVE THERAPIES FOR THE TREATMENT OF COPD

Lung volume reduction surgery (LVRS)

LVRS may effect a significant improvement in respiratory clinical benefit and functioning for some patients. At present within the UK, the selection criterion for this procedure is specific and offered in few secondary centres. However, LVRS does not appear to alter the mortality rate of COPD. The surgery removes functionless areas in lungs of patients with COPD and thereby improves the mechanics of breathing by reducing thoracic volumes (Cooper *et al.* 1996). An adaptation of this procedure to deliver surgical isolation of some of the more damaged regions of the lung via a bronchoscopic approach is outlined by Toma and Geddes (2003). It is interesting to note that there is now some consideration being given to the development of more specific approaches of LVRS in terms of the treatment of COPD.

Lung transplantation

This is a possible method that might be used to improve COPD respiratory function; however the procedure has significant operative mortality rate associated with it. The long-term sequela requiring the taking of medication to reduce the probability of rejection should not to be discounted or minimised when arriving at a decision to undertake the treatment.

CARING FOR COPD PATIENTS IN
THE COMMUNITY SETTING

As previously discussed, the majority of care received by patients with COPD will be carried out in the community. This has become the accepted pattern following the granting of the necessary funding required to ensure the provision of the health needs of their local community, to the Primary Care Trusts (PCTs). The change not only makes economic sense: more importantly it funds a better basis for the provision of patient care. It is expected that those patients with COPD will find that the local community care GP-based practice is now able to respond quicker to their changing medical demands.

The almost universal use of electronic databases in Primary and Secondary Care Centres has the potential to improve efficiency and maximise the range of services these care centres can now offer all patients. Not least are the benefits they can now provide for patients with COPD. The records of patients that have been compiled and held independently in the Primary and Secondary Care Centres become almost instantly and mutually accessible for clinical purposes. Consultations can be arranged; adverse effects of medication notified; advice requested and given; and agreed protocols documented – all possible without the previous delays that could be so critical to the patient.

Larger general practices often employ practice nurses who specialise in care for chronic respiratory diseases such as asthma and COPD. Once a diagnosis of COPD has been made, whether by a nurse or a GP, it is accepted practice to place such patients upon the practice register for repeated review of their condition. This is known as 'call and recall' and forms a pivotal role in the care of chronic illness.

This 'call and recall' system once fully in operation encourages the beginning of a working relationship, within which all the points and issues relating to the disease could be discussed.

This will be important to both the health professional and the patient with COPD, since the fostering of such a therapeutic relationship will provide the basis of continuing support for the patient and family.

In conclusion it must be stressed that COPD is a progressive incurable disease that has significant physiological, psychological and emotional effects upon the patient and the family. The financial cost of providing care for those with COPD is a substantial drain on the resources allotted to the NHS and welfare state while any 'carer's allowances' are probably rarely capable of reimbursing either the financial or the emotional costs to the patient and family.

Treatment at present focuses upon reducing the impact and severity of COPD to the patient by providing smoking cessation information; medication to alleviate symptoms; and rehabilitation therapy to promote physical and emotional wellbeing.

COPD exacerbations have a significant effect upon the patient and the rate of disease progression, but rapid and appropriate treatment will significantly improve the recovery following an exacerbation (NICE 2004).

The health professional should ensure that all the key issues are addressed in the management of COPD and that an open, honest therapeutic relationship with the patient and family is developed to encourage the discussion of those issues of particular relevance to the patient.

SUMMARY
❏ COPD is a progressive, incurable disease.
❏ Early diagnosis and commencement of appropriate management will improve patient quality of life.
❏ Management of COPD focuses upon maintaining functional health status of the patient and reducing/minimising the incidence of COPD exacerbations.
❏ Symptomatic pharmacological treatment with inhaled bronchodilators and inhaled steroids will provide improved morbidity for those with COPD.
❏ Prevention of acute exacerbations will improve patient's health status.

❏ Acute exacerbations can be treated at home or in the secondary care setting.

❏ Choice of location for the treatment of COPD exacerbations is clearly outlined in the NICE 2004 COPD guidelines.

❏ Acute exacerbations require rapid patient assessment, including the need for supplemental oxygen therapy, nebulisation of medication and antibiotic therapy.

❏ Discharge from secondary care setting should be a collaborative multidisciplinary approach with appropriate follow-up ensured in primary care.

❏ Early and appropriate pulmonary rehabilitation will help patients to maintain their functional health status.

❏ Smoking cessation will have a positive effect upon lung function.

❏ Nutritional advice and assessment has been proven to aid in the management of COPD.

❏ Deterioration of COPD for some patients will necessitate the commencement of long-term oxygen therapy (LTOT).

REFERENCES

American Thoracic Society (1995) Standards for the diagnosis and care of patients with COPD. *American Journal of Respiratory and Critical Care Medicine* **152** (5, pt 2): S77–S121.

Ashcroft J (2003) Supporting smoking cessation in the general practice setting. *Airways Journal* **1**: 8–9.

Barnes PJ (2000) Mechanisms in COPD: differences from asthma. *Chest* **117** (2 Suppl.): 10S–4S.

Bellamy D (2003) How to differentiate asthma from COPD in primary care. *Airways Journal* **1**: 10–14.

Boe J, Dennis JH, O'Driscoll RR *et al.* (1984) The prevalence and determinants of nutritional changes in COPD. *Chest* **88**: 558–563.

Braun SR, Dixon RM, Keom NL *et al.* (1984) Predictive clinical value of nutritional assessment factors in COPD. *Chest* **85** (3): 353–357.

Britton M (2003) The burden of COPD in the UK: results from the Confronting COPD survey. *Respiratory Medicine* **97** (Suppl. C): S71–S79.

BTS COPD Guidelines Group of Standards of Care Committee of the BTS (1997) BTS Guidelines for the Management of COPD. *Thorax* **52** (Suppl. 5): S1–S28.

BTS (2002) Guidelines on non-invasive ventilation in acute respiratory failure. *Thorax* **57**: 192–211.

Burge PS, Calverley PMA, Jones PW, Spencer S, Anderson JA, Maslen TK. (2000) Randomised double blind, placebo controlled study of fluticasone propionate in patients with moderate to severe COPD. The ISOLDE trial. *British Medical Journal* **320**: 1297–1303.

Campfield LA, Smith FJ, Bun P (1996) The OB protein (leotin) pathway – a link between adipose tissue mass and central neural networks. *Hormone Metabolism Research* **38**: 619–632.

Chavannes N (2004) The necessity for spirometry in the primary care management of COPD. *Primary Care Respiratory Journal* **13**: 11–14.

Clark NM, Becker MH, Janz NK *et al.* (1991) Self management of chronic disease by older adults. *Journal of Ageing and Health* **3** (1): 3027.

Collins CM (2003) Nutrition and the COPD patient. *Airways Journal* **1**: 94–97.

Cook D, Guyatt G, Wong E *et al.* (2001) Regular versus as needed short-acting inhaled beta-agonist therapy for chronic obstructive pulmonary disease. *American Journal of Respiratory and Critical Care Medicine* **163**: 85–90.

Cooper JD, Lefrak SS (1999) Lung-reduction surgery: 5 years on. *Lancet* **353** (Suppl. 1): 26–27.

Cooper J (2001) Partnerships for successful self management: the living with long-term illness report. Long Term Medical Conditions. (Lill) project, Alliance London.

Creutzberg E (2003) Leptin in relation to systemic inflammation and regulation of the energy balance. *European Respiratory Monograph* **24**: 56–67.

Dahl R, Greefhorst LA, Nowark D *et al.* (2001) Inhaled formoterol dry powder versus ipratropium bromide in COPD. *American Journal of Respiratory Critical Care Medicine* **164** (5): 778–784.

Department of Health (2001) *The expert patient: a new approach to chronic disease management for the 21st century.* The Stationery Office, London.

Doll R, Peter R, Wheatley K *et al.* (1994) Mortality in relation to smoking: 40 years' observations on male British doctors. *BMJ* **309** (6959).

Donaldson GC, Seemungal TA, Bhourmik A, Wedzicha JA (2002) Relationship between exacerbation frequency and lung function decline in COPD. *Thorax* **57**: 847–852.

Donner CF, Decramer M (2003) Pulmonary rehabilitation. *European Respiratory Monograph* **24**: 1–6.

Donahue JF, van Noord JA, Bateman ED *et al.* (2002) A 6 month placebo controlled study comparing lung function and health status changes in COPD patients with tiotropium or salmeterol. *Chest* **122** (1): 47–55.

ERS: Siafakas NM, Vermeire P, Pride NB *et al.* (1995) Optimal assessment and management of COPD. The European Respiratory Society Task Force. *European Respiratory Journal* **8** (8): 1398–1420.

Gibbons D, Bartley J (2003) A study to investigate high readmission rates for COPD. *Professional Nurse* **19** (4): 208–212.

Gibbons D, Hamilton J, Maw G, Telford J (2001) Developing a nurse led service for COPD patients. *Professional Nurse* **16** (4): 1035–1037.

GOLD: Pauwels RA, Buist AS, Claverley PM, Jenkins CR, Hurd SS (2001) Global strategy for the diagnosis, management and prevention of chronic obstructive pulmonary disease. NHLB1/WHO Global initiative for chronic obstructive lung disease (GOLD) workshop summary. *American Journal of Respiratory Critical Care Medicine* **163** (5): 1256–1276.

Gravil JH, Al-Rowas OA, Cotton MM *et al.* (1998) Home treatment of acute exacerbations of chronic obstructive pulmonary disease by an acute respiratory assessment service. *Lancet* **351** (9119): 1853–1855.

Griffiths H, Jordan S (2002) Corticosteroids: implications for nursing practice. *Nursing Standard* **17** (12): 43–53.

Halpin DMG (2001) *COPD.* Mosby, Philadelphia.

Halpin DMG (2004) Bronchodilators in COPD: the long and short of it. *Airways Journal* **2** (1): 30–32.

Holman H, Larig K (2000) Patients as partners in managing chronic disease. Partnership is a pre-requisite for effective and efficient health care. *BMJ* **320** (7234): 526–527.

Hugli O, Fitting JW (2003) Alterations in metabolism and body composition in chronic respiratory diseases. *European Respiratory Monograph* **24**: 11–22.

Hunter AMB, Cavey MA, Larg HW (1981) The nutritional status of patients with chronic obstructive pulmonary disease. *American Review of Respiratory Disease* **96**: 556–565.

Jones PW, Bosh TK (1997) Quality of life changes in COPD patients treated with salmeterol. *American Journal of Critical Care Medicine* **155** (4): 1283–1289.

Jones WPJ, Ferro-Luzzi A, Waterlow JC (1988) Definition of chronic energy deficiency in adults. *European Journal of Clinical Nutrition* **42**: 969–981.

Kline Leidy N, Ozbolt JG, Swass MAP (1990) Psychophysiological processes of stress in chronic physical illness: a theoretical perspective. *Journal of Advanced Nursing* **15**: 478–486.

Lacasse Y, Guyatt GH, Goldskin RS (1997) The components of a respiratory rehabilitation programme. *Chest* **111**: 1077–1088.

Lansen R (2003) Effects of inflammation on skeletal muscle. *European Respiratory Monograph* **24**: 35–45.

Lau AC, Yam LY, Poon E (2001) Hospital re-admission in patients with acute exacerbations of COPD. *Respiratory Medicine* **95** (11): 876–884.

Lopez AD, Murray CC (1998) The global burden of disease, 1990–2020. *Natural Medicine* **4** (11): 1241–1243.

Lorig KA, Sobel DS, Stewart AL *et al.* (1999) Evidence suggesting that a chronic disease self management program can improve health status while reducing utilisation and costs: a randomised trial. *Medical Care* **37** (1): 5–14.

Medical Research Council (MRC) Committee on the Aetiology of Chronic Bronchitis. (1965) Definition and classification of chronic bronchitis for clinical and epidemiological purposes. *Lancet* **1**: 775–779.

Mosier K, Renvall MJ, Ransdell JW, Spinder AA (1996) The effects of theophylline on metabolic rate in chronic obstructive lung disease patients. *Journal of the American College of Nature* **15**: 403–407.

Nicassio PM, Smith W (eds) (1995) *Managing chronic illness. A biopsychosocial perspective.* Psychological Association, Washington DC.

NICE (2002) *Guidance on the use of nicotine replacement therapy (NRT) and bupropion for smoking cessation.* Guidance no. 38.

NICE (2004) COPD national guideline on management of chronic obstructive pulmonary disease in adults in primary and secondary care. *Thorax* **59** (Suppl. 1): 1–232.

NICE (2004) COPD National Office for National Statistics (2000) *Mortality statistics: Cause, 1999.* DH2 (no. 26). London, HMSO.

Office for National Statistics. (2000) Mortality statistics: Cause, 1999. DH2 (no. 26). HMSO, London.

Peperall K, Rudolf M, Pearson M, Diggle J (1997) *Asthma in General Practice* **5**: 29–30.

Percival J (2004) The art of helping people to stop smoking. *Airways Journal* **2** (1): 18–21.

QUIT (2004) Quit: helping smokers to stop. *Airways Journal* **2**: 1–50.

Ram FSF, Lightowler JVVJ, Wezicha JA (2003) Non-invasive positive pressure ventilation for the treatment of respiratory failure due to exacerbations of COPD. *Cochrane Review Issue 3.* Oxford, Cochrane Library.

Scanlon PD, Connett JE, Waller LA, Altose MD, Bailey WC, Buist AS (2000) Smoking cessation and lung function in mild to moderate COPD. The lung health study. *American Journal of Respiratory Critical Care Medicine* **161** (2, pt 1): 381–390.

Schiffelers S, Blaak E (2003) Fat metabolism in chronic respiratory disease. *European Respiratory Monograph* **24**: 34–45.

Schols AMWJ, Burg J (2003) Efficacy of nutritional intervention in COPD. *European Respiratory Monograph* **24**: 142–152.

Schols AMWJ, Slangen J, Volovics L, Wouters EFMM (1998) Weight loss is a reversible factor in the prognosis of COPD. *American Journal of Respiratory Care Medicine* **157**: 1791–1797.

Seamark DA, Williams S, Timon S *et al.* (2001) Home or surgery based screening for chronic obstructive pulmonary disease (COPD). *Primary Care Respiratory Journal* **10** (2): 30–33.

Selby C (2002) *Respiratory medicine: an illustrated colour text.* Churchill Livingstone, Edinburgh.

Sestini P, Renzami E, Robinson S, Poole P, Ram FS (2000) Short-acting beta two agonists for stable COPD. Cochrane Review. *Cochrane Database Systematic Review 3.*

Sethi JM, Rochester CL (2000) Smoking and chronic obstructive pulmonary disease. *Clinics in Chest Medicine* **21** (1): 67–86, viii.

Siafakas NM, Vermeire P, Pride NB *et al.* (1995) Optimal assessment and management of COPD The European Respiratory Society Task Force. *European Respiratory Journal* **8** (8): 1398–1420.

Silverman EK (2001) Genetics of chronic obstructive pulmonary disease. *Novartis Foundation Symposium* **234**: 45–58; discussion 58–64.

Sin DD, Tu JV (2000) Outpatient antibiotic therapy and short term mortality in elderly patients with chronic obstructive pulmonary disease. *Canadian Respiratory Journal* **7**: 466–471.

Smit HA, Grievink L, Tabak C (1999) Dietary influences on chronic obstructive lung disease and asthma: a review of the epidemiological evidence. *Proceedings of the Nutrition Society* **58**: 309–319.

Toma TP, Geddes DM (2003) COPD: is there anything new around the corner? *Airways Journal* **1**: 26–29.

Vincken W, van Noord JA, Geofhorst AP *et al.* (2002) Improved health outcomes in patients with COPD during one year's treatment with tiotropium. *European Respiratory Journal* **19** (2): 209–216.

West R, McNeill A, Raw M (2000) Smoking cessation guidelines for health professionals: an update. Health Education Authority. *Thorax* **55** (12): 987–999.

Whittle P (2004) Response to: the necessity for spirometry in the primary care management of COPD. *Primary Care Respiratory Journal* **13**: 15–16.

Zuwallack R (2003) The effects of nutritional depletion on health status. *European Respiratory Journal* **24**: 132–141.

Nebulisers and Inhalers

4

In cases of respiratory illness the prompt delivery of medication to alleviate the symptoms and potentiate the healthy function of the lungs is of prime importance. The anatomy and physiology of the lungs provide an ideal route for the delivery of the medication, especially if its target is the respiratory system itself. The surface area of the adult lungs is about $100\,m^2$ and that interface is supplied with an underlying extensive and prolific blood supply. Such a system provides the key requirements for the effective delivery of localised and systemic medication. Inhalation is thus widely regarded as not only being the most convenient and practical but also the best route of administration for drugs in the treatment of airway obstruction (Burnell *et al.* 2001). Targeting the lungs for the delivery of medication dates back to the 19th century, when volatile inhalation anaesthetics were administered for their systemic effects and hand-operated nebuliser devices were also introduced for medicinal use (Benson & Prankerd 1998).

The aims of this chapter include:
❏ Outlining how inhalation medication therapy is delivered to the lungs.
❏ Explaining how the common inhaler devices operate, and noting particularly their advantages and disadvantages.
❏ Nursing implications involved when considering selection of inhaler devices and patient education.
❏ Principles of nebuliser therapy.
❏ Patient issues with regard to encouraging their concordance with medication, selection of inhaler device and education requirements.

PRINCIPLES OF DRUG DELIVERY TO THE LUNGS

Most drug administration to the lungs is designed to produce a local effect (Brown 2004), for example in the treatment of asthma or cystic fibrosis. The most common method for the precise targeting of the lungs with appropriate medication is via inhalation of the drug, usually with the medication dispersed in the form of an aerosol. Devices that have been designed to aid/provide this delivery mechanism fall into two broad classes: nebulisers and inhalers. The principles of their operation will be considered in this chapter. However they all utilise the properties of aerosols to deliver their medication.

Medication inhaled as an aerosol exerts its effect only if it is correctly and appropriately placed within the lungs, a process known as deposition. This presents a challenge to the pharmaceutical industry in the design of pulmonary preparations (Aulton 1990). For deposition to occur, medication inhaled into the lungs has to have the properties of an aerosol defined as 'a dispersion of solid or liquid particles (typically $<5\,\mu m$) in a gas' (Aulton 1990). Aerosols in pulmonary medication are composed of particles with a range of sizes; particles less than $3\,\mu m$ will penetrate the alveoli, while those that range between $3–5\,\mu m$ distribute uniformly throughout the lung (Benson & Prankerd 1998).

Particle deposition within the lungs is dependent upon several mechanisms (Brown 2004):

- **Inertial impaction.** This occurs when a particle carried in a gas stream has enough momentum (the product of its mass and velocity) to continue in the direction that it is initially travelling, even if the gas stream bearing it along changes direction. The particle will thus impact with whatever is in front of it rather than continue along in the flow of gas. This form of deposition tends to occur in the uppermost regions of the respiratory tract and it mainly affects the larger sized particles that will thus fail to reach the lower regions of the lung.
- **Sedimentation.** This is as a result of gravitational forces acting on the particles and is an important mechanism deter-

mining the deposition in the lower airways of particles of between 0.5 and 3.0 µm. Gravitational forces are not however as important a factor in determining the movement of the smaller sized particles within the lungs.

- **Diffusion**. The smallest drug particles will collide with the gas and water molecules that surround them, causing the particles to exhibit Brownian movement. Those particles that collide with the lung surface are being constantly adsorbed, thereby establishing a diffusion gradient. Diffusion towards the walls of the respiratory tract is particularly important with the smaller particles less than 0.5 µm.

The **solvent and propellants** used in the design of the medication delivery device also have an effect upon the deposition of the medication particles. That variable together with patient anatomy, breathing patterns and other factors all have a significant effect. Consequently the design of inhalers and nebulisers has to evaluate and take all these factors into consideration.

Understanding the principle of particle deposition provides clarity and logic to the protocol detailing how inhalers should be used. **Breathing the aerosol in slowly and deeply** reduces the impaction occurring in the upper airways, the buccal cavity and pharynx, allowing the medication to travel onwards towards the smaller airways (Benson & Prankerd 1998). **Breath holding following the inhalation of the aerosol** gives time for sedimentation and diffusion to occur (Anon 2000). If the breath is not held most of the smaller medication particles will be exhaled and consequently the therapeutic deposition of the medication is unlikely to have been achieved.

Case study: Richard Hunter, Part 1

Richard Hunter aged 72 has, for a number of years, had a respiratory illness. He has been prescribed and used inhalers to provide symptomatic relief and therapeutic treatment of his respiratory symptoms for over six years. However in the past year he has found that he needs to use more and

Continued

---

more of his prescribed medication, with a diminished return in respect of relief of his symptoms. Mr Hunter sought the advice of his GP, who referred him to the practice nurse for a review of his respiratory illness. Mr Hunter attended an appointment with the practice nurse who during the interview asked him to demonstrate how he used his inhaler medication.

Mr Hunter took from his pocket his standard pressured metered dose inhaler and placed it to his lips. He pressed the canister button to dispense the medication from the device and there appeared from his nose and lips a fine aerosol mist.

What immediate information can you obtain from the above case study?

Mr Hunter is experiencing an increase in his respiratory symptoms; this could be due to his disease progressing in severity or changing in aetiology and thereby requiring a different treatment. He also quite clearly cannot use his inhaler device correctly to ensure that lung deposition of the medication designed to relieve his respiratory symptoms occurs.

TYPES OF INHALER

The most common and cheapest type of inhaler device is a pressurised metered dose inhaler (pMDI). Most of the inhaled medications to treat respiratory illness are available in this type of inhaler. If this device is used well and timely the deposition of the medication to the lungs can be as high as 20% of the dose dispensed (Anon 2000, Roche Products Ltd 2002, Brown 2004).

How to use a pMDI

(Palen *et al.* 1997; see Fig. 4.1.)

1. Shake the inhaler.
2. Remove dust cap from the mouthpiece.
3. Exhale fully.

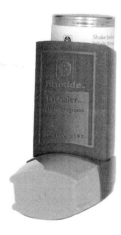

Fig. 4.1 pMDI. With permission from Allen and Hanburys.

4. Place to the lips and form a tight seal around the device.
5. Press the canister as inhalation begins.
6. Breath in slowly and deeply.
7. Hold breath for at least 5 seconds, ideally for 10 seconds.
8. Expire.
9. Replace dust cap.

If a second dose of the medication is required, wait at least 20 seconds and then repeat steps 1–9 above.

Alternative devices based upon the standard pressurised metered dose inhaler exist. This group includes Autohalers™ and Easi-breathe™ devices. These devices dispense their medication automatically upon the inspiration of those using the device. These inhalers remove from the user of the device the necessity to press the canister at the start of inspiration, thereby reducing the high level of co-ordination and manual dexterity required to use the pMDIs. These devices are slightly more expensive than pMDIs.

Dry powder inhalers (DPIs)

These create an aerosol when the patient inhales through them. A sufficient flow rate is required to disperse the drug into small particles, and depending upon device these flow rates can vary from 15–60 L min^{-1} (Brown 2004). The inspiration pressure exerted by the patient generates the flow rate. Deposition into the lungs is about 30% of the dose (Brown 2004). Diskhalers^{TM}, Turbohalers^{TM} (Fig. 4.2), Clickhalers^{TM} and Accuhalers^{TM} are examples of DPIs. There are some variations between the various devices available and differences in their precise method of usage. Although there may be differences in the details the general principles of their operation are very similar.

As an example the operation of an Accuhaler^{TM} is as follows:

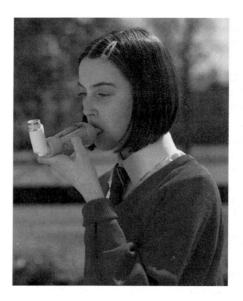

Fig. 4.2 Able Spacer (in use). With permission from Clement Clarke International.

1. Open device by sliding case back. This automatically triggers the counter which counts down from 60–1. The last few numbers are written in red to warn the user that the inhaler will shortly be empty.
2. Exhale fully.
3. Place mouthpiece to lips and inhale through mouth.
4. Hold breath for a count of ten (*circa* ten seconds).
5. Expire.
6. Shut device; this primes the device and thus upon the next opening of the Accuhaler the delivery of the medication is assured.

If a second dose of the medication is required, repeat steps 1–6 above.

Table 4.1 provides information on the range of inhalers available and their advantages and disadvantages. Note, this table should be read in conjunction with the current British National Formulary or equivalent reference to obtain updated, correct and accurate information on the range of medication available in each type of inhaler device.

CHOICE OF INHALER DEVICE
This will depend upon the following criteria (Goodman *et al.* 1994, Palan *et al.* 1997, BTS 2003, NICE 2004):

- Patient ability to use device.
- Patient's preference.
- Stage of respiratory disease.
- The necessity for adjuncts that either simplify the use of inhaler device or increase its performance, e.g. large volume spacer or small volume spacer.
- Type of medication prescribed.
- Cost.
- Range of other inhaler devices that patient may already have.

The 2003 BTS guidelines and the NICE 2004 guidelines both recommend that the use of pMDIs should be augmented by the use of large volume spacer devices. These devices are designed

Table 4.1 Range of inhalers available.

Name of inhaler	Advantages	Disadvantages	Principal medication available
pMDI	Cheap Small Fits spacer devices	Requires high level of co-ordination Not suitable for young and older people No method of determining how much medication remains in canister	Salbutamol Terbutaline Salmeterol Beclometasone (formally Beclometasone) Budesonide Fluticasone Ipratropium bromide Sodium cromoglycate
Easi-breathe	Removes co-ordinating inspiration with pressing canister. Suitable for young and older people. Low inspiration pressure required	Relatively expensive. Bulkier than a standard pMDI No method of determining how much medication remains in canister	Salbutamol Beclometasone Sodium cromoglycate
Autohaler	Small Primes itself with displacement of lever	Not all medication available in this type of inhaler device Relatively expensive. Bulkier than a standard pMDI No method of determining how much medication remains in canister	Salbutamol Beclometasone
Diskhaler	Dose counter available Low inspiratory pressure required	Not all medication available in this type of inhaler Requires high level of dexterity Needs regular cleaning	Salbutamol Salmeterol Beclometasone Fluticasone

Table 4.1 *Continued.*

Name of inhaler	Advantages	Disadvantages	Principle medication available
Accuhaler	Counter facility provides information on how many doses left Small, easily portable. Moisture proof	More expensive than pMDI Not all respiratory medication available in this type of device	Salbutamol Salmeterol Fluticasone
Clickhaler	Counter indicates how many doses remain in inhaler Small	Not all respiratory medication available in this product type. More expensive than pMDI Affected by a moisture rich environment	Salbutamol Beclometasone
Handi-haler		Patients will need another type of inhaler for relief of respiratory symptoms, since only tiotropium available in this device	Tiotropium
Turbohaler		Not suitable for young children, due to high inspiratory pressure required	Terbutaline Eformoterol Fumarate Budesonide

to increase the amount of medication deposition that occurs in the lungs. Without the use of large volume spacers less than 20% of the dose is deposited in the lungs (see previous text). With the use of a large volume spacer this can increase to between 40 and 60%. Consequently the use of large volume spacers is now strongly advocated in all situations when a pMDI is prescribed for patient use.

Certainly the use of large volume spacers should be consistently and strongly recommended to all children and older people using the pMDI. They should be convinced that the value of ensuring a higher dose deposition outweighs any apparent social disadvantages. The use of a large volume spacer is as follows.

Use of large volume spacer

The large volume spacer is supplied in two parts that lock in place when fitted together. Small children may require the fitting of a facemask as a further aid. These children's facemasks vary in size, but babies have to be supplied with their own designed large volume spacer 'babyhaler'.

There are two recognised methods of using large volume spacers:

Method 1 (tidal breathing)

This procedure is suitable for all users, but it is found to be especially useful for children and older people. This is because it requires minimal effort upon inspiration and is easy to remember.

Shake the pMDI and then place the nozzle so that it fits securely in the manifold hole within the large volume spacer. Place the mouthpiece of the large volume spacer into the mouth and form a tight seal around it. Press the canister and then inhale and exhale five times; this is known as tidal breathing. Holes exist in the mouthpiece of the large volume spacer which allow the egress of the expired air into the surrounding atmosphere thus eliminating the risk of re-breathing expired air with a high concentration of carbon dioxide. A further valve controls the operation of the large volume spacer. This valve opens upon inspiration allowing the inhalation of the medication. It closes upon expiration. The use of a large volume spacer ensures that the larger particles produced in the aerosol remain within the large volume spacer thus the impaction of the medication is reduced within the buccal cavity and pharynx. The smaller particles that are inhaled will rapidly progress into the smaller airways.

The use of a large volume spacer has much to commend it. Most importantly it removes the need for good co-ordination between inspiration and the finger depressing the canister button. The failure to ensure good co-ordination is one of the major reasons why the use of the pMDI on its own is not always the most efficient method of therapeutic drug delivery.

Method 2: hold breath before expiration

For the second method of using the large volume spacer, proceed as above but instead of using the method known as tidal breathing, depress the canister and then take a deep breath from the mouthpiece and hold breath for a count of ten (*circa* ten seconds) before expiration. This method is most suitable for adults.

The large volume spacer has a limited life span of between 6 and 12 months, depending upon how often the large volume spacer is used. These devices gradually build up an electrostatic charge due to the deposition of the medication on the wall surfaces within the large volume spacer. Eventually this charge renders these devices as useless adjuncts in the delivery of the medication. Routine care includes the washing of the large volume spacers in warm soapy water, but they should then be left to air dry to minimise the build up of electrostatic charge.

There are other problems associated with the use of large volume spacers, for example they are quite bulky and thus not easily portable in the school bag. Their size also tends to attract attention to its user.

An increase in the lung deposition of the medication can also be attained when smaller spacer devices, such as the 'Aerochambers', are used in conjunction with the pMDI devices. However the improvement in lung deposition is not as high as that achieved by the use of large volume spacers. They have a similar lifespan to that of the large volume spacers and should be washed in the same method.

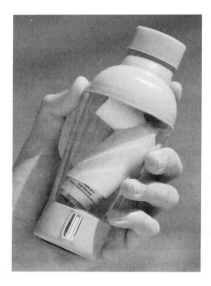

Fig. 4.3 Able Spacer chamber. With permission from Clement Clarke International.

Figure 4.3 shows an example of a small volume spacer, in this case an able chamber.

Dry powder inhaler devices (DPIs) are particularly suitable for those patients who have difficulties achieving the manual dexterity required to use pMDIs. However, not all dry powder devices operate by the same mechanism and as already discussed the flow rate required to achieve inspiration of the medication varies from device to device. For example the Accuhaler requires lower inspiratory pressures than the Turbohaler (Burnell *et al.* 2001). Equipment exists which can help in the decision-making process as to which inhaler device may be the most suitable for the patient, i.e. 'In Check Dial™'; however it provides only a guide to the decision-making process (Tovar & Gums 2004).

NURSING IMPLICATIONS

The importance of the choice of inhaler device should not be underestimated. It is essential that the patient is consulted and allowed choice in this issue since this will aid in maintaining concordance with the therapeutic regime prescribed. The treatment of a respiratory illness is often of a long duration; it may even extend throughout the patient's lifetime. The self-motivation and self-discipline needed to continue the day upon day compliance with the prescribed medication regime is thus an important factor in ensuring that the maximum response and benefits are derived. Empowering patients, especially in the choice of inhaler device, is an important first step in aiding them to live up to such a demanding concordance.

Inhaler technique

Nurses should be aware of the common types of inhaler devices and how they should be used. Ad hoc opportunistic assessment of patient's ability to use inhalers should be siezed. The patient's 'inhaler technique' can reveal common easily rectifiable problems which can then be corrected to enable a more advantageous use of the device and an improvement in the patient's respiratory symptoms (Haro-Estarriol *et al.* 2002, Palen *et al.* 1997). Such opportunities could and do occur on any ward or hospital unit and these occasions are not restricted to those patients who are admitted primarily as a result of respiratory symptoms. Health care professionals who routinely interact with respiratory patients should always assess patients' inhaler technique. BTS (2003) guidelines on the management of asthma suggest that every time a patient with asthma has contact with a health professional their inhaler technique should be assessed. This was endorsed subsequently by NICE (2004) and they advocate that a regular review of inhaler technique should be carried out and appropriately documented.

Research has found that many patients who have inhaler devices throughout Europe are unable to use them well (Haro-Estarriol *et al.* 2002). Palen *et al.* (1997) had established that 40% of the researched subjects did not perform all the essential inhaler manoeuvres correctly. The findings broadly reflect the results they obtained from the whole range of inhalers available (Turbohalers, Diskhalers, Rotahalers, pMDIs, etc.). The correct use of pMDIs scored the lowest rating, with only 24% of those using such devices shown as able to use them correctly. This deficiency in technique was further substantiated by Broeders *et al.* (2003) who found that pMDIs were so badly used that even after instruction there was little improvement in patients' inhaler technique. Broeders *et al.* suggested that pMDIs alone should not be used in certain client groups, such as those patients with severe COPD. This reservation has become a major factor to consider among some health professionals who have raised similar concerns about their effective use with children (Goodman *et al.* 1994). A smaller percentage of adolescents were found unable to use prescribed pMDIs correctly (Francis 2001) but in this group instruction did significantly reduce the number who were unable to employ the correct technique. The improvement noted seemed to be largely sustained when re-tested after several months. A significant proportion of young adults, middle-aged and older people have also been shown to employ defective techniques when using pMDIs.

Any failed assessment of inhaler technique must be followed by corrective measures. Education and information is still probably the most cost effective course of action, but it must be sustained to ensure that either excellent inhaler technique by the patient continues, or poor inhaler technique improves. If no improvement is noted in inhaler technique consideration must be given to altering the type of inhaler device.

Education for patients

Much research has been undertaken on the importance of education for patients and on the methods found to be the most effective ways of disseminating information (Palen *et al.* 1997). Group instruction, the use of video demonstrations and individual instruction have all improved patient use of their inhaler device (Palen *et al.* 1997). This process remains primarily within the province of nursing, since nurses often develop good therapeutic relationship with both patients and their families. But even in the acute clinical situations, for example in A & E units, any time taken to teach patients how to use inhaler devices will reduce the probability of their re-admission due to exacerbation of symptoms. Any improvement is marked by an improvement in the patient's quality of life.

The National Respiratory Training Centre (NRTC) based in Warwick strongly advocate that not only are patients told how to use their inhaler device, they are also demonstrated its correct use. This recommendation is further supported by BTS (2003), and NICE (2004). In many hospitals the routine demonstration of inhaler technique is usually undertaken by respiratory specialist nurses. Other nurses may be unable to undertake this role since they do not have ready access to placebo inhalers and other training devices. However, all health professionals should be familiar with the correct use of the common types of inhalers. This has in the past not been the case in either primary or secondary care settings, with many health professionals having little or even inaccurate knowledge concerning how to use inhaler devices (Hanania *et al.* 1995). There thus exists a pool of health professionals who are not only unable to successfully teach patients how to use inhaler devices, but are also unaware of the latest developments. With the increasing demand by health professionals for courses and information on the use of inhalers this is perhaps a diminishing problem.

Patients and their families should be given written information that succinctly summarises the key issues and actions necessary in the correct use of their inhaler device. The use of written information alone can improve patients' use of inhaler devices (Hernandez *et al.* 2004), but it is better practice to demonstrate the use of the inhaler device and reinforce this with written information. Many manufacturers produce these leaflets, for example GlaxoSmithKlein produce many product-related leaflets illustrating the correct use of pMDIs and Easibreathe devices (see Fig. 4.4). Similar leaflets are produced by the manufactures of dry powder devices (see Fig. 4.5) illustrating the use of Turbohalers.

action asthma
This is where it starts

How to use your aerosol inhaler properly

• Remove the mouthpiece cover and check the mouthpiece inside and outside to see that it is clean

• Shake the inhaler well

• Hold the inhaler upright as shown above with your thumb on the base, below the mouthpiece. Breathe out as far as is comfortable and then...

PLEASE TURN OVER

• Place the mouthpiece in your mouth between your teeth and close your lips firmly around it, **but do not bite it**

• Just after starting to breathe in through your mouth, press down on the top of the inhaler to release the medication while still breathing in steadily and deeply

• Hold your breath, take the inhaler from your mouth and your finger from the top of the inhaler. Continue holding your breath for as long as is comfortable

action asthma
This is where it starts

• If you are to take a second puff keep the inhaler upright and wait about half a minute before repeating steps 2 to 6
• After use always replace the mouthpiece cover to keep out dust and fluff

important

Do not rush Stages 3, 4 and 5. It is important that you start to breathe in as **slowly** as possible just before operating your inhaler. Practise in front of a mirror for the first few times. If you see "mist" coming from the top of the inhaler or the sides of your mouth you are not doing it properly and you should start again from Stage 2.

If your doctor has given you different instructions for using your inhaler, please follow them carefully.
Tell your doctor if you have any difficulties.
TESTING YOUR INHALER If you have not used your inhaler for a week or more release one puff into the air to make sure that it works.

To learn more about asthma, visit www.actionasthma.co.uk

Fig. 4.4 Patient information leaflet: use of PMDIs. Reproduced with permission from GlaxoSmithKlein.

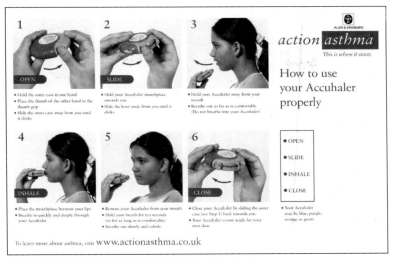

Fig. 4.5 Patient information leaflet: use of accuhalers. Reproduced with permission from GlaxoSmithKlein.

Case study: Richard Hunter, Part 2

The practice nurse upon observing Mr Hunter's inhaler technique responded appropriately and spent some time demonstrating to him how to use the inhaler correctly. Mr Hunter was then assessed again following his observation of the practice nurse; this time there was no obvious aerosol escape from his nose and mouth (the major cause of this effect is pressing the canister but not simultaneously inspiring). However Mr Hunter still had some problems using his inhaler correctly and the practice nurse felt it appropriate to introduce the use of a large volume spacer to aid in his use of his inhaler.

Continued

Mr Hunter was given information to read, followed by a demonstration by the practice nurse on the correct use of the large volume spacer. He then had his ability to use the large volume spacer assessed.

Mr Hunter then left his general practice with clear printed instructions on how and when to use his inhalers together with his prescription for a large volume spacer. He was also asked to keep among other documentation a symptom diary that would be reviewed by his GP the following week. This follow-up appointment was necessary because Mr Hunter had been prescribed a modification to his treatment following the review undertaken by the practice nurse.

The GP found that Mr Hunter did not have severe symptoms following the initiating of Mr Hunter into the use of a large volume spacer. His medication was reviewed but no significant changes were made. Mr Hunter reported that once again the medication was working.

Comment

It had been a number of years since Mr Hunter had had his use of his inhaler device reviewed. As with many things in life, as time had progressed he found that using his inhaler took time and effort and had adapted his use of the inhaler to suit himself. This focused review directly addressing and explaining how the device worked and reinforced by providing a simple adjunct, had not only improved Mr Hunter's quality of life but may, by reducing his symptoms, have even prevented his admission to hospital.

The correct use, cleaning and maintenance of inhalers and spacer devices should be clearly explained to patients and families. Dry powder devices should ideally be kept out of rooms that regularly have moist atmosphere, i.e. kitchens and bathrooms. Although many of these devices contain a desiccate to prevent the medication becoming too moist for delivery, it is best to try to reduce or avoid exposure to moisture. Shaking dry powder devices that contain a desiccant is not a reliable method to ascertain whether the inhaler device is empty or not. These devices will always rattle even when empty of medication due to the presence of the desiccant.

Pressurised metered dose inhalers containing pressurised gas, should not be exposed to extreme temperatures and must be kept away from naked flames.

NEBULISERS

Traditionally these devices have been recommended and used in cases of severe respiratory distress when the patient has been unable to 'breath hold' for a sufficient period of time to allow the therapeutic deposition of their medication to be given via an inhaler device. However this view is now being challenged. Increasingly research is demonstrating that the use of a large volume spacer and a pMDI can deliver a sufficient deposition of bronchodilator and inhaled steroid medication to effectively replace the need for nebulisation therapy (Eiser *et al.* 2001a, Numata *et al.* 2002).

Numata *et al.* (2002) provided evidence that even in acute respiratory distress in an Accident and Emergency setting it could take less than 6.5 minutes to successfully teach patients how to use a large volume spacer with pMDI and gain therapeutic relief from bronchodilators. In a few instances some patients required nebulisation only once to relieve their immediate respiratory distress. When the symptoms had abated enough to allow sufficient patient concentration to undertake instruction, the use of pMDIs and the large volume spacer was used thereafter for the administration of bronchodilator therapy. Brocklebank *et al.* (2001) found in a systematic review that there was no benefit in the use of nebulisers over pMDIs and large volume spacers. However they did suggest that further research should be undertaken to determine the economic implications and to elucidate whether the clinical findings would still hold in the community setting.

Eiser *et al.* (2001b) found that both nebuliser therapy and pMDI with large volume spacers allowed patients with severe end-stage COPD to improve their respiratory functioning as

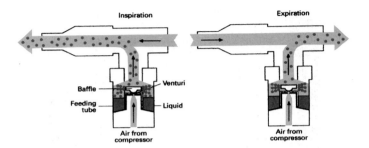

Fig. 4.6 How nebulisers work; from BTS guidelines. Reproduced with permission from BMJ Publishing Group (BTS 1997).

measured by a six-minute walking test and residual volume. They concluded that in the community setting nebulised therapy provided little benefit over the use of pMDIs with large volume spacers.

In England and Wales nebulisers and compressors are not available on the NHS (BNF 2004); however some are available on form GP10A in Scotland.

There are three main types of nebuliser (see Chapter 5):

- Jet nebuliser.
- Ultrasonic nebuliser.
- Adaptive aerosol delivery system.

Jet nebulisers

Jet nebulisers consist of a reservoir that holds the required medication and a system for generating a Venturi effect (see Chapter 5) when compressed air or oxygen is forced through a small hole in the nebuliser unit. The oxygen or compressed air is used to break up the solutions or suspensions of medication into droplets for inhalation (Brocklebank *et al.* 2001). Figure 4.6 illustrates how nebulisers work. Larger particles are returned to the reservoir after colliding with part of the nebuliser and only the smaller particles are released to form the mist inhaled by the patient.

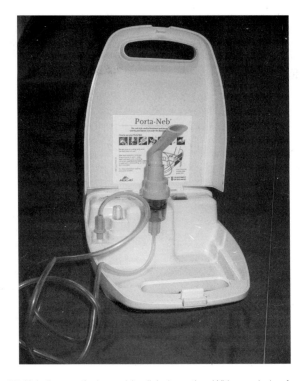

Fig. 4.7 Nebuliser routinely used in clinical practice. With permission from the National Respiratory Training Centre.

Figures 4.7 and 4.8 illustrate nebulisers routinely used in clinical practice.

A rate of gas flow of between $6-8\,L\,min^{-1}$ is required to produce an aerosol where 50% of the particles are less than $5\,\mu m$. The propellant gas is either compressed air or oxygen. Air is often used in the home environment, primary care practice and in many cases where type II respiratory

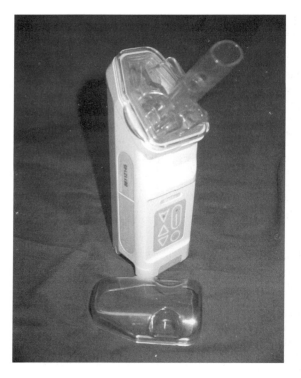

Fig. 4.8 Nebuliser routinely used in clinical practice. With permission from the National Respiratory Training Centre.

failure is involved. Domiciliary oxygen cylinders cannot provide an adequate flow to power jet nebulisers. Oxygen is used as the propellant gas in situations of type I respiratory failure.

If patients have type II respiratory failure requiring maintenance oxygen therapy, then it is possible to deliver bronchodilator therapy via a nebuliser while continuing oxygen therapy via nasal cannulae. However this is quite arduous for the patient and the oxygen delivery tubing plus the facemask can become quite claustrophobic.

Ultrasonic nebulisers

Ultrasonic waves are passed through the medication to generate aerosol droplets. Such ultrasonic generators will nebulise larger volumes than jet nebulisers and are usually quieter. However they cost more than the jet nebulisers and are often not as robust.

Adaptive aerosol delivery systems

These are designed to utilise the patient's individual breathing pattern to maximise the therapeutic delivery of the medication by delivering the aerosol at suitable periods of inspiration but not during expiration (Nikander 1997).

Nebulisation therapy

All nebulisers currently available will retain a residual volume of medication left within the storage chamber when the nebulisation is complete. This volume varies from device to device and is quite clearly stated on the product information leaflets. Most residual volumes are between 0.5 and 2.5 mL. It is important that all health professionals involved in care of patients undergoing treatment with this equipment are reminded of this residual volume. Patients should not have to endure nebulisation therapy for long periods of time in a vain attempt to deliver all the medication left within the chamber.

The smaller the residual volume the smaller the fill volume required to commence the nebulisation. The nebuliser chamber must be filled to a minimum fill volume in order to achieve adequate aerosol delivery of suitable particle size to allow lung deposition. This fill volume can be as little as 2.5 mL if residual volume is less than 1 mL, or lie between 4 mL and 5 mL if the residual volume is greater than 1 mL. Checking the information enclosed with the nebuliser is an important part of the preparation required to ensure correct therapeutic medication delivery for the patient.

The time taken for nebulisation varies, depending upon fill volume of chamber; flow rate of driving gas; and the patient's ability to comply with treatment. Nebulisation time should be between 5 and 10 minutes (Murphy 2001) for bronchodilators; however some medication may be required to be given over a longer period of time. Any extension to the time increases the risk that patients find themselves unable to cope with the equipment, noise, facemasks, etc. and thus cease complying with the medication. The importance of clear, effective patient and family information should not be underestimated in these situations, since this may be persuasive and thereby increase patient compliance by alleviating their anxieties.

The patient interface device for the delivery of nebulisation therapy is either a mouthpiece or a facemask. A mouthpiece is the interface device of first choice, since it provides a higher level of drug deposition than facemasks and reduces the claustrophobic sensation that some patients experience when wearing facemasks. However the mouthpiece relies upon the patient having the ability to hold it in place while breathing through their mouth. This may not be possible for the very young or older population and they may benefit from the use of a facemask. The facemask must be tight fitting and this can cause irritation to the face especially during long periods of nebulisation therapy. Patient choice should be the main driving factor in choice of interface device.

The British Thoracic society (2003) recommends that the use of nebulisers in chronic persistent asthma should be considered carefully, taking into consideration the following factors:

- Review of diagnosis.
- Airflow obstruction must be significantly reversed by bronchodilators without unacceptable side effects.
- Use of inhaler device has been checked and ensured adequate.
- Increased dose of bronchodilator via hand held inhaler device has been tried for at least two weeks.
- Patient compliance with all medication has been assured.

If the need for a nebuliser at home is established after considering the above criteria, then a two-week trial of nebulisation therapy should be undertaken. If this indicates that there is a need for a home nebuliser the following steps should be carried out:

- Patient should have clear instructions on how to use nebuliser and associated equipment.
- Be instructed not to treat acute attacks at home without seeking medical help first.
- Receive a rolling education programme.
- Have regular follow-up, including peak flow monitoring.

SUMMARY

❏ Inhalation of medication is a common and convenient method of delivering respiratory medication.

❏ Hand-held inhaler devices are the most frequently used method of delivering respiratory medication to the lungs.

❏ Patient-related factors, including inhaler technique rate and depth of inspiration, anatomy and physiology of the lungs will influence the amount of medication deposited in the lungs.

❏ The use of adjuncts such as large and small volume spacer devices will increase the lung deposition of respiratory medication.

❏ Patient education and preference are crucial in selecting the type of inhaler device, and in considering any alteration in inhaler device.

❏ Regular review and follow-up are required to ensure that patient inhaler technique remains adequate.

❏ Oxygen or compressed air drives nebulisers.

❏ Selection and use of nebulisers in a hospital setting will depend upon type of medication, patient preference and duration of nebulisation therapy.

❏ The use of nebulisers at home should be limited and based upon specific clinical need, ensuring regular review of the patient by appropriate health professionals.

REFERENCES

Anon (2000) Inhaler devices for asthma. *Drug Therapy Bulletin* **38** (2): 9–14.

Aulton ME (1990) *Pharmaceutics: the science of dosage from design.* Churchill Livingstone, London.

Benson HA, Prankerd RJ (1998) Optimisation of drug delivery – pulmonary drug delivery. *Australian Journal of Hospital Pharmacy* **28:** 18–23.

Bernard-Bonnin AC, Stachenko S, Bonnin D *et al.* (1995) Self management teaching programs and morbidity of pediatric asthma: a meta analysis. *Journal of Allergy and Clinical Immunology* **95:** 34–41.

British Medical Association (2004) *British National Formulary (BNF).* Royal Pharmaceutical Society of Great Britain, London.

British Thoracic Society (1997) Current best practice for nebuliser treatment. *Thorax* **52** (Suppl. 5): S1–S28.

British Thoracic Society, Scottish Intercollegiate Guidelines Network, National Asthma Campaign, British Association for Accident and Emergency Medicine, General Practice in Airways Group, Royal College of Paediatrics and Child Health, Royal College of Physicians of London (2003) British Guideline on the Management of Asthma. A national clinical guideline. *Thorax* **58** (Suppl. 1): i1–i94.

Brocklebank D, Ram F, Wright J *et al.* (2001) Comparison of the effectiveness of inhaler devices in asthma and chronic obstructive airways disease: a systematic review of the literature. *Health Technology Assessment* **5** (26): 1–149.

Broeders ME, Molema J, Hop WC, Folgering HT (2003) Inhalation profiles in asthmatics and COPD patients: reproducibility and effect of instruction. *Journal of Aerosol Medicine* **16** (2): 131–141.

Brown R (2004) Drug delivery systems 2. Pulmonary and parenteral formulations. *Airways Journal* **2** (1): 43–46.

Burnell PKP, Small T, Doig S, Johal B, Jenkins R, Gibson GJ (2001) Ex-vivo product performance of Diskus™ and Turbohaler™ inhalers using inhalation profiles from patients with severe chronic obstructive pulmonary disease. *Respiratory Medicine* **95:** 324–330.

Clark C (1998) Concordance is not a PC term. *Pharmaceutical Practice* March: 83.

Davies DS (1975) Pharmacokinetics of inhaled substances. *Postgraduate Medical Journal* **51** (Suppl. 7): 69–75.

Eiser NM, Phillips C, Wooler PA (2001a) Does the mode of inhalation affect the bronchodilator response in patients with severe COPD? *Respiratory Medicine* **95:** 476–483.

Eiser N, Angus K, McHale S (2001b) The role of domiciliary nebulisers in managing patients with severe COPD. *Respiratory Medicine* **95** (4): 265–274.

Francis C (2001) School clinics for adolescents with asthma. *Professional Nurse* **16** (8): 1281–1284.

Gallefoss F, Bakke PS (2000) Impact of patient education and self management on morbidity in asthmatics and patients with chronic obstructive pulmonary disease. *Respiratory Medicine* **94**: 279–287.

Goodman DE, Israel E, Rosenberg M, Johnston R, Weiss ST, Drazen JM (1994) The influence of age, diagnosis, and gender on proper use of metered dose inhalers. *American Journal of Respiratory Critical Care Medicine* **150** (5 pt 1): 1219–1221.

Hanania NA, Wittman R, Keston S, Chapman KR (1995) Medical personnel's knowledge of and ability to use inhaling devices. Metered-dose inhalers, spacing chambers and breath actuated dry powder inhalers. *Chest* **105** (1): 111–116.

Haro-Estarriol M, Lazaro Castaner C, Marin Barneuvo C *et al.* (2002) Usefulness of teaching how to manage the pressurized canister and the Turbohaler system in hospitalized patients. *Archivos de Bronconeumologia* **38** (7): 306–310.

Hernandez L, Abellan AJ, Martinez CJ, Nicolas BA (2004) Written information on the use of aerosols in COPD patients. Can we improve their use? *Atencion Primaria* **33** (1): 6–10.

Murphy S (2001) In: Esmond G (ed.) *Respiratory nursing*. Churchill Livingstone, Edinburgh.

Newman SP, Clarke SW (1983) Therapeutic aerosols. 1: Physical and practical considerations. *Thorax* **38**: 881–886.

Newman SP, Millar AB, Leonard-Jones TR *et al.* (1984) Improvement of pressurised aerosols inhaled through extension devices. *American Review of Respiratory Disease* **124**: 317–320.

NICE (2004) Chronic obstructive pulmonary disease. *Thorax* **59** (Suppl. 1): 1–232.

Nikander K (1997) Adaptive aerosol delivery: the principles. *European Respiratory Review* **7** (51): 385–387.

Numata Y, Bourbeau J, Ernst P, Duquette G, Schwartzman K (2002) Teaching time for metered dose inhalers in the emergency setting. *Chest* **122** (2): 498–504.

Palen J, Klien JJ, Kerkhoff AHM, Herwaarden CLA, Seydel ER (1997) Evaluation of the long term effectiveness of three instruction modes for inhaling medicines. *Patient Education and Counseling* **32**: S87–S95.

Premaratne UN, Sterne JAC, Marks GB *et al.* (1999) Clustered randomised trial of an intervention to improve the management of asthma: Greenwich asthma study. *British Medical Journal* **318**: 1251–1255.

Roche Products Ltd (2002) *Summary of product characteristics, Pulmozyme*. Roche Products Ltd.

Tovar JM, Gums JG (2004) Monitoring pulmonary function in asthma and COPD: point of care testing. *Annals of Pharmacotherapy* **38** (1): 126–133.

Oxygen Therapy

5

Oxygen therapy is commonly administered in both primary and secondary care settings (Jevon & Ewens 2001, Dunn & Chisholm 1998). Its use is almost considered 'routine' in many clinical situations, for example, post-anaesthetic care units, intensive therapy units, accident and emergency departments and by paramedics treating patients in respiratory distress. Although it is now administered by all health care professionals including junior doctors, oxygen therapy continues to remain one of the most misunderstood treatments (Smith & Poplett 2002). The subject thus requires a more careful and detailed consideration (Ashurst 1995, Simmons & Simmons 2004).

Oxygen is classified pharmacologically as a prescription only medication under the Medicines Act 1968 and thus should always be prescribed for use with a specified patient. Some clinical areas have a generic prescription or 'blanket policy' in which oxygen therapy can be commenced as required without a specific individual prescription; for example some accident and emergency departments. However, many clinical areas do not have such policies and in these areas oxygen should always be prescribed for each individual requiring this treatment. The only exceptions to this general rule are life-threatening situations in which the use of oxygen therapy can be commenced immediately to maintain life.

The aims of this chapter are to review:

❑ The key principles associated with the administration of oxygen therapy.

❑ How the common oxygen delivery devices work, considering their advantages and disadvantages.

❑ The principles and practice of humidification therapy.

❏ The assessment of patients for the commencement and cessation of oxygen therapy.
❏ The medical implications of long-term oxygen therapy (LTOT).
❏ The principles of both non-invasive ventilation and invasive ventilation.

The gas known as 'oxygen' was discovered by Joseph Priestly in the late 18th century. Shortly after its discovery it was used to treat patients in hospital with acute and chronic respiratory failure. It was noted that this provided some relief of the respiratory distress these patients were experiencing, providing a reduction of breathlessness and improved mobility (Dunn & Chisholm 1998).

Oxygen is essential for the survival of the cells of the body. Breathing and respiration together in normal fit and healthy people ensure that the correct concentration of oxygen is maintained within the tissues (please refer to Chapter 1). Oxygen concentration is maintained between 12 and 14 kPa in arterial blood, allowing adequate gas exchange to occur to support cellular respiration (Guyton & Hall 2000). If the oxygen concentration falls outside these upper and lower bounds then there are consequential effects upon the tissues of the body, the duration and concentration of the altered arterial oxygen level determining their severity.

A high concentration of oxygen within the arterial bloodstream can result in oxygen toxicity and consequential blindness, cellular membrane damage and progression into adult respiratory distress syndrome (ARDS) which can in some cases lead to death (Bateman & Leech 1998). Too low a concentration results in a fall in aerobic cellular respiration that would have a devastating effect upon the tissues of the body and could also result in death. Consequently the human body is adept at ensuring that the ideal concentration of oxygen is maintained within the arterial blood, adjusting many factors including those observable changes in the rate and depth of inspiration to ensure homeostasis. However there are times when despite the efforts of the body to maintain homeostasis, the oxygen concentration within the arterial blood falls, a condition known as hypoxaemia. In such cases, it is then often necessary to consider intervention and provide oxygen therapy. The presence of hypoxaemia in clinical situations is often considered to indicate the existence of respiratory failure, which in the majority of cases will require intervention.

Blood loss or acute infection are among the many causes of hypoxaemia; however it is most commonly associated with oxygenation failure and/or ventilatory failure. Table 5.1 illustrates a few of the major causative reasons for hypoxaemia.

Respiratory failure is subdivided into two classes: type I and type II (BTS 2002). Type I respiratory failure is distinguished clinically in cases when arterial blood gas analysis (see Chapter 8) indicates that hypoxaemia is present but there is no associated hypercapnia (increase in carbon dioxide concentration). Type I respiratory failure usually occurs for example in acute asthma attacks, chest trauma, and pneumonia. Type II respiratory failure is distinguished by the presence of hypoxaemia and hypercapnia upon arterial blood gas analysis. This condition may be found to be present during exacerbations of COPD, in grossly obese patients, and in those displaying debilitating neuromuscular weakness.

Table 5.2 illustrates the possible range of arterial blood gas analysis in both normal, type I and type II respiratory failure.

Table 5.1 Major causes of hypoxaemia.

- **Oxygenation failure:** ventilation perfusion mismatch is the commonest cause of oxygenation failure within the lungs. This is when there is either adequate perfusion (by the blood) but inadequate ventilation within regions of the lung (result of airway obstruction), or when there is adequate ventilation but inadequate perfusion (such as pulmonary embolus).
- **Ventilatory failure:** for example hypoventilation can be due to effects of medication on the respiratory centre, i.e. use of opiates, barbiturates; chest trauma; Guillain–Barré syndrome; muscular dystrophy affecting the respiratory muscles; upper airway obstruction (Woodcock & Partridge 1996).

Table 5.2 Arterial blood gas values.

Arterial blood analysis	Normal	Type I respiratory failure	Type II respiratory failure
pH	7.35–7.45	7.35–7.45	7.35–7.35 or <7.35
PaO_2	12–14 kPa	<8 kPa	<8 kPa
$PaCO_2$	4.6–6.0 kPa	4.6–6.0 kPa	>6 kPa
SaO_2	95%+	<92%	<92%

Table 5.3 defines some of the common respiratory terms used when assessing the need for oxygen therapy.

INDICATIONS FOR THE USE OF OXYGEN THERAPY
Oxygen therapy is used to correct:

- Type I respiratory failure (hypoxaemia only).
- Type II respiratory failure (hypoxaemia and hypercapnia).
- Palliative relief of shortness of breath (Esmond & Mikelsons 2001).

Type I respiratory failure
Type I respiratory failure associated with hypoxaemia requires that the patient receives oxygen therapy supplied at a concentration that is sufficient to correct the hypoxaemia. This may vary from patient to patient and can, for example in cases of acute severe asthma, pneumonia or heart failure, require oxygen levels as high as 60–100% to be administered in order to correct the hypoxaemia. Repeated arterial blood gas measurements are not usually necessary in type I respiratory failure, once initial measurements have indicated that there is no hypercapnia (rise in carbon dioxide). Peripheral oxygen saturation measurements via pulse oximetry together with detailed clinical assessment of the patient is usually sufficient to assess the progress of the patient with oxygen therapy. It is important to note that oxygen therapy should be reduced as the clinical condition of the patient improves.

Table 5.3 Common respiratory assessment terms.

Hypoxia:	decreased availability of oxygen to the tissues to allow normal cell function (Dunn & Chisholm 1998).
Normoxia:	suitable level of oxygen available to tissues, allowing normal tissue function.
Hyperoxia:	greater level of oxygen available to tissues than is required to allow normal function.
Hypoxaemia:	insufficient oxygen concentration within the arterial blood (Esmond & Mikelsons 2001).
Hypoventilation:	decreased rate of breathing resulting in too little air entering the respiratory tract to allow adequate respiration to occur.
Hyperventilation:	increased rate of breathing above the metabolic demands of the body resulting in hypocapnia.
Tachypnoea:	a high rate of breathing, >20 breaths per minute (Torrance & Elley 1997).
Bradypnoea:	a low rate of breathing, <12 breaths per minute (Torrance & Elley 1997).
Dyspnoea:	difficulties in breathing.
Hypercapnia:	increased carbon dioxide concentration outside normal limits within the arterial bloodstream.
Orthopnoea:	a condition in which the person must stand or sit upright to breathe comfortably.
Apnoea:	absence of breathing.
Hyperpnoea:	high rate of breathing.
Cheyne–Stokes:	respiratory pattern = periods of apnoea alternate with periods of hyperpnoea. Causes include left ventricular failure, cerebral injury and sometimes occurs in patients at the end stages of their life.
Kussmaul breathing:	(air hunger) deep rapid respirations due to stimulation of the respiratory centre in the brain caused by for example metabolic acidosis, ketoacidosis or renal failure.
pH:	the negative common logarithmic concentration of hydrogen ions $pH = -\log_{10}[H^+] = \log_{10}[1/H^+]$ where $[H^+]$ is expressed in moles per litre.
PaCO$_2$:	partial pressure of oxygen in arterial blood: normal range 4.7–6 kPa.
SaO$_2$:	arterial blood oxygen saturation, usually measured directly upon arterial blood gas analysis.
SpO$_2$:	peripheral blood oxygen saturation, often measured indirectly via pulse oximetry.

Type II respiratory failure

Type II respiratory failure is often associated with COPD, gross obesity, or chronic neuromuscular weakness. Patients who display this syndrome have in the past caused the most concern during the administration of oxygen therapy. Type II respiratory failure frequently develops over a significant period of time, during which the carbon dioxide concentration within the blood stream may have increased above the normal range (hypercapnia).

In normal, fit healthy individuals it is the rise in carbon dioxide concentration within the bloodstream that initiates inspiration (see Chapter 1, 'The hypoxic drive', p. 8). In patients displaying type II respiratory failure, the rise in carbon dioxide concentration within their bloodstream will have a diminished role in triggering inspiration. Consequently in these cases inspiration is often initiated when there is a fall in oxygen concentration to below its normal bounds. Thus intervention in response to hypercapnia could prove counterproductive. For example, the administration of oxygen therapy would increase the oxygen concentration within the patient's arterial blood and this may result in reducing the rate and depth of breathing. This induced phase of hypoventilation will, by reducing the rate of carbon dioxide loss from the lungs, further compound the already increased carbon dioxide level within the patient's arterial blood and thus exacerbate the problem of hypercapnia. To avoid triggering this sequential chain of events there must be careful consideration of how to undertake the administration of oxygen therapy in type II respiratory failure. When oxygen therapy is used it is usually commenced at low levels of 24–28%, and increased as patient assessment dictates. Arterial blood gas analysis is essential in type II respiratory failure and should be repeated at judicious intervals, titrating oxygen therapy against arterial blood carbon dioxide concentration (Bateman & Leech 1998). Peripheral pulse oximetry is not sufficient as the sole monitoring of oxygen therapy in type II respiratory failure, however it should still be used in this case as an adjunct to clinical decision-making.

PALLIATIVE USE OF OXYGEN

Chapter 3 outlined the benefits that acute end-stage COPD patients experience following the administration of oxygen therapy. Oxygen therapy can benefit other patients where distress is associated with shortness of breath. For example those patients with lung cancer will describe a subjective benefit gained by short periods of oxygen therapy, the length and frequency of the therapy being dictated by the patient's needs.

PATIENT ASSESSMENT

Accurate, timely and appropriate assessment of patients with respiratory conditions is crucial. The assessment must provide: information concerning respiratory function; an evaluation of the patient condition; and time for the monitoring and adjustment of any equipment used in intervention therapy. The respiratory assessment of patients should consider the following issues and all pertinent observations and signs should be appropriately documented.

Effectiveness of breathing

Chest movement should be equal, symmetrical and bilateral (Jevon & Ewens 2001). Consideration should also be given to the depth of inspiration, type of breathing and frequency (respiration rate). Chest auscultation will also indicate the presence of bilateral breath sounds and should be audible in all lung zones (Bennett 2003).

Indicators of work-load of breathing

Fit, well and healthy subjects at rest breathe quietly with minimal effort. Noisy respiration, increased respiration rate, the use of accessory muscles, to breathe e.g. abdominal muscles, sternomastoid muscles indicate that greater effort is required to breathe (Clutton-Brock 1997).

Every observation must be placed in the context of any prior activity recently undertaken. A reference to the activity, time and location should form part of the annotation required. Thus if an individual has just run 400 m and is out of breath it is considered 'acceptable and normal' to use all the accessory muscles and increase the respiration rate. However this would not be an acceptable consequence for an individual who is usually healthy, fit and well but now finds himself out of breath when walking slowly on level ground for 4 m. The presence of extraneous factors, such as constriction imposed by clothing, carrying heavy loads, climbing stairs, etc. would also immediately and subconsciously be taken into account by the observer but may require to be recorded. Severe respiratory distress is indicated if patients cannot talk, complete sentences, eat or drink. Breathlessness may cause patients to alter their lifestyle, reduce the distance they can walk, cease climbing stairs, avoid certain activities, and alter the position they sleep in. Information on such changes should be obtained and documented.

Adequacy of ventilation
Failure to achieve a satisfactory level of ventilation may be indicated by adverse changes in a number of key functions:

- Breathlessness.
- Heart rate. A breathless person can experience tachycardia initially but in cases of extreme hypoxia this can alter to bradycardia.
- Skin colour. Pallor and the presence of cyanosis.
- Mental status. Confusion and agitation often occur in periods of hypoxia.

Peripheral pulse oximetry and arterial blood gas analysis provide information concerning the adequacy of ventilation (Jevon & Ewens 2001).

General appearance
The presence of finger clubbing can indicate pulmonary or vascular disease. The condition is indicated by the loss of nail bed angle, increased curvature of the nail and swelling of the terminal part of the digit. Anxiety and fear are common emotions of breathless patients; an unkempt appearance may indicate difficulties in general physical care due to breathlessness.

Social and medical history

It is important to note whether the patient has any previously diagnosed respiratory or cardiovascular conditions; past and current medication; and whether the patient already has oxygen therapy at home. Family history of respiratory disease should also be considered, for example, asthma has a strong genetic link and is often a familial condition.

Occupational history

This should be considered against exposure to known respiratory irritants, e.g. coal dust, flour.

Patient assessment should be repeated as required by the clinical condition of the patient (Torrance & Elley 1997). For example an individual in acute respiratory failure (type I) should have high flow oxygen therapy commenced as soon as possible and the effects of the treatment continuously monitored.

A patient who is unable to talk is unlikely to be able to provide significant useful social and medical history; however if relatives can be contacted they may well supply useful information. Once the patient's condition improves more detailed assessment may continue and social and medical history be completed (Ahern & Philpot 2002).

COMPLICATIONS OF OXYGEN THERAPY

There are many problems associated with oxygen therapy. However the commonest are:

- Retention of carbon dioxide.
- Respiratory acidosis (Guyton & Hall 2000).
- Reduction in the hypoxic drive to breath (Smith 2004).
- Mucosal drying and mucociliary dysfunction (Bourke 2003).
- Dehydration of respiratory secretions and sputum retention (Pilkington 2004).
- Atelectasis (lung collapse); since high inspired oxygen concentrations can reduce surfactant production (a substance which stabilises alveolar membrane and reduces surface tension) (Jevon & Ewens 2001).

- Oxygen toxicity particularly likely after respiring for more than 48 hours a gas mixture containing a high concentration oxygen. This may subsequently progress into adult respiratory distress syndrome that has a high associated mortality (Bateman & Leech 1998).
- Fire risks.

Some of these complications can be reduced by the careful and appropriate selection of the oxygen delivery system and the use of adjuncts such as humidification systems (Esmond & Mikelsons 2001). However it is the responsibility of all who provide care for patients requiring oxygen therapy to be aware of the possible complications and repeat patient assessments, considering the results against the possible complications of oxygen therapy.

NURSING RESPONSIBILITIES
- Support, reassure and educate patients and their families to gain their compliance with the administration of oxygen therapy (Sheppard & Davis 2000).
- Promote and ensure patient safety during oxygen therapy, following local policies, guidelines and national protocols. The mandatory rule that there must be no smoking on any ward where oxygen therapy is being given should be rigorously enforced. Clear instructions on the matter must be given personally to patients and relatives, preferably while explaining the reasons for such an embargo. The rule extends to cover any areas where oxygen therapy is occurring, or where oxygen storage devices such as portable oxygen cylinders are being stored.
- Consideration of the administration of oxygen therapy should be alongside the principles of the administration of medications (UKCC 2000), and nurses should be familiar with all the points outlined in Table 5.4.

Regular oral hygiene is essential since mucosal drying is a known side effect of oxygen therapy. If possible patients should be encouraged to have a high oral fluid intake and appropriate fluids must always be available.

Table 5.4 Nursing responsibilities in the administration of oxygen (UKCC 2000).

1. Know the therapeutic uses of oxygen, the normal doses, side effects, precautions, contra-indications and hazards.
2. Be certain of the identity of the patient receiving the oxygen.
3. Ensure that the prescription is unambiguous and written clearly. This includes the percentage of oxygen required, rate of flow, duration of oxygen therapy, need for humidification and type of oxygen delivery system, for example nasal cannulae or face mask (Bell 1995).
4. Consider the method, timing and commencement of oxygen therapy against the background of the patient's condition and other co-morbidities.
5. Contact the prescriber of the oxygen therapy, or other appropriate person, if contra-indications to the prescribed oxygen are discovered: if the patient develops a reaction; if the patient refuses oxygen therapy and/or if the patient assessment indicates that oxygen therapy is no longer required.
6. Make a clear, accurate and immediate record when oxygen is administered, withheld or refused by patient. Ensuring that all written information is pertinent, legible and signed. If this task is delegated it is the registered nurse's responsibility to ensure that this is carried out.
7. Monitor vital signs, observing patient for any change in respiratory distress or symptoms.
8. Record time, date, method of delivery, rate of flow and concentration of oxygen. Assess the patient's rate and depth of breathing, colour, mental state, and respiratory pattern at commencement of oxygen therapy.

Reproduced with permission and modified from Jevon P, Ewens B (2001) Assessment of a breathless patient. *Nursing Standard* **15** (16): 48–53.

Assessment of the patient should be frequent and this includes checking to ensure that the oxygen therapy device is correctly and comfortably positioned and delivering the correct prescribed oxygen therapy. The oxygen tubing should also be checked since there are cases reported of patients becoming hypoxic when this tubing has become blocked in both anaesthetic and ward use (Penney *et al.* 2000). If humidification therapy is also required then this should be scrutinised to ensure that it is correctly fitted and that the water level is not below that recommended by the manufacturers. Humidification apparatus that introduces heat into the oxygen therapy should be carefully checked to ensure that the inspired gas is not above the mandated temperature. Hot gases can severely burn the respiratory tract (Jevon & Ewens 2001).

Breathless patients often require help with activities such as washing, dressing and mobilisation. It is important not to overwhelm the patient with too many of these tasks and ensure that timely help and assistance is given. In many cases a step-by-step approach is adopted and this often meets patients' needs while reducing episodes of breathlessness (Jevon & Ewens 2001, Bennett 2003). As the patient's condition improves the ability to undertake these tasks can be an effective measurement of their improvement and act as a patient-centred goal to work towards.

SELECTION OF OXYGEN DELIVERY SYSTEMS FOR THE ADMINISTRATION OF OXYGEN THERAPY

For spontaneously breathing patients this is based upon a consideration of the following factors (Jevon & Ewens 2001, Bennett 2003, Vines *et al.* 2000):

- Type of respiratory failure.
- Rate and depth of patient's inspiration and expiration.
- Oxygen concentration prescribed.
- Need for humidification.
- Likely duration of oxygen therapy.
- Patient preference/tolerance (Sasaki *et al.* 2003).
- Location of patient whether at home or in hospital.
- Cost.

All oxygen delivery systems consist of an oxygen source (e.g. cylinder, concentrator), oxygen flow meter (see Fig. 5.1), oxygen tubing and a device which directly interfaces with the patient to deliver the oxygen (e.g. nasal cannulae, facemask) (Jevon & Ewens 2001, Bennet 2003).

There are two categories of oxygen delivery devices for those patients who are spontaneously breathing: **fixed performance devices** and **variable performance devices**.

Fixed performance devices

These include in their delivery circuit a venturi adaptor that supplies oxygen to the patient and allows for the mixing of the oxygen with air drawn into the system through holes in the adaptor (see Fig. 5.1).

Operation of Venturi Valve

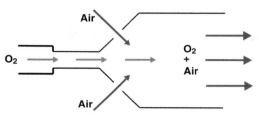

Fig. 5.1 Operation of Venturi valve.

Patients receive a concentration of oxygen therapy that is independent of their rate and depth of breathing. The size of the inlet holes that allow mixing of oxygen with air varies with each type of adaptor to alter the oxygen concentration inspired by the patient. Such fixed performance masks have large holes in them to allow the egress of air and thereby reduce the risk of rebreathing a significant concentration of carbon dioxide. This makes these devices ideal for use in type II respiratory failure. However, some studies have indicated that in cases when oxygen therapy is required above 40% then Venturi systems may not deliver the required concentration of oxygen, with the patients receiving between 5 and 10% lower oxygen concentration than would be indicated by the venturi adaptor selected (Iooss *et al.* 1997).

Variable performance devices
These include nasal cannulae, Hudson delivery systems and any other systems that do not incorporate a Venturi adaptor (Esmond & Mikelson 2001, Bennett 2003). These systems will deliver a percentage of oxygen that is dependent upon the patient's rate and depth of inspiration, and are thus suitable for those patients that do not require accurate percentage oxygen to be delivered. They are thus most suitable for patients in type I respiratory failure.

These devices may also have to be employed when 'patient choice' must take precedence over clinical preference. Some patients will not accept or tolerate fixed performance masks and in such cases it is possible, even if not desirable, to use variable performance systems such as nasal cannulae to deliver oxygen therapy. Nasal cannulae may also be substituted for fixed performance delivery systems for those patients requiring oxygen therapy whilst eating and drinking.

Non-rebreathe masks

These masks allow the delivery of high concentrations of oxygen approximately 95% at flow rates of $12\,L\,min^{-1}$ or higher (AHA 1997). The reservoir bag contains a one-way valve to prevent exhaled air entering the oxygen reservoir bag. On inhalation, the one-way valve opens to direct oxygen from a reservoir bag into the mask; thus the patient breathes air from the reservoir bag only. In addition, one-way valves are located on the side ports to prevent room air entering the mask. A tight seal is required, which can be difficult to maintain and uncomfortable for patients.

These devices are thus only suitable for short-term therapy (Vines *et al.* 2000). The reservoir bag should be able to expand freely and should not be kinked or in any way constricted. Oxygen flow rates should be sufficient to keep the bag inflated.

Use of humidification systems

Humidification systems aim to prevent or reduce some of the complications associated with the delivery of supplemental oxygen (Fell & Boehem 1998). Specifically the use of humidification will reduce or prevent:

- Respiratory tract mucosal drying.
- Dehydration of respiratory secretions and subsequent sputum retention.
- Atelectasis (lung collapse).
- Increased risk of infections.
- Pain associated with a dry respiratory tract and retained secretions.
- Blocking of tracheostomy tubes.

The need for humidification should be assessed for each individual patient. It is used mainly in situations in which one or more of the following conditions apply:

- Requires a high flow rate delivery of oxygen greater than $4 L min^{-1}$ (Bateman & Leech 1998).
- Oxygen therapy to be carried out for more than 4 hours.
- A respiratory tract infection has occurred.
- There are difficulties clearing sputum; producing thick purulent secretions.
- Predisposed respiratory condition exist: for example cystic fibrosis which will increase the risk of the complications associated with the delivery of oxygen therapy.
- Requiring CPAP (continuous positive airways pressure).
- Has a tracheostomy.

Humidification systems are for convenience described as being either active or passive systems. The active systems add water and may add heat to the inspired gas. These humidifiers mainly operate by forcing a gas (usually air and/or oxygen) through a water storage device to produce a fine water mist. The passive systems, for example HMEs (heat and moisture exchangers), rely upon the warm moist air exhaled by the patient to humidify the inspired gas. The majority of the airborne particles should be in the range of 0.5–1.0 microns in order to reach the peripheral airways.

Table 5.5 illustrates the range of humidification systems available in clinical practice, and Table 5.6 shows the range of oxygen masks available.

NON-INVASIVE AND INVASIVE VENTILATION
In severe respiratory failure, either type I or type II clinical situations can occur in which it is necessary to consider further adjuncts to aid patients in the work of breathing other than just additional oxygen delivery. These usually fall into two classes, invasive and non-invasive ventilation.

The term **non-invasive ventilation (NIV)** is applied to the clinical use of ventilatory support using a non-invasive patient interface, for example nasal mask or full facemask. Such

Table 5.5 Range of humidification systems available.

Name of humidification device	Advantages	Disadvantages
HME (Hydro-Trach T) also known as a Swedish Nose	Used on tracheostomy tubes.	Oxygen connected via additional tubing. Delivers unpredictable oxygen concentrations that vary with the oxygen flow rates and the patient's rate and depth of inspiration.
Nebuliser with saline	Useful for short-term, concentrated humidification. Ideal for patients with sputum retention.	Delivers unpredictable oxygen concentrations that vary with oxygen flow rate, and patient's rate and depth of inspiration.
Bubble humidifier	Brings oxygen to ambient levels of humidity. Used with: nasal cannulae; medium concentration masks; and higher concentration Venturi masks (>35%). Normally used unheated.	Should not be used with low concentration Venturi masks i.e. 24–28%, nasal cannulae. May not provide adequate humidification.
Humidifier nebuliser	Attached directly to oxygen flowmeter and connected to an aerosol mask via Flex tube. Allows precise oxygen concentration of 28–35–40–60% (24% is possible via an adaptor). High humidification output. Fits most popular, standard sterile water bottles.	
Pass-over humidifier e.g. Devilbiss ultrasonic humidifier	Normally used in intensive care settings. Can be used with fixed concentration masks via elephant tubing and a humidification cup.	Expensive.

Line drawings reproduced with permission of *Intersurgical®*.

Table 5.6 Range of oxygen masks available.

Name of oxygen delivery device/patient interface	Advantages	Disadvantages
Variable performance facemask	• Suitable for type I respiratory failure. • Delivers oxygen concentrations between 35 and 60%. • Low cost product.	• Cannot deliver more than 60% oxygen concentration. • Should not be used with flow rates. $<5\,L\,min^{-1}$ as 'rebreathing' may occur. • Delivers unpredictable concentrations that vary with oxygen therapy and patient's ventilation pattern. • Impractable for long-term use. • Not suitable for patients with COPD. (Jeffrey & Warren 1992)
Nasal cannulae	• Suitable for patients with both type I and type II respiratory failure. • Delivers oxygen concentrations between 22 and 35%. • Comfortable and well-tolerated, reduces experience of claustrophobia. • Patients can eat and drink with nasal cannulae in situ. • No rebreathing. • Low cost product. (Bazuaye *et al.* 1992)	• Cannot be used for medium/high oxygen concentrations (>40%). • Not suitable for patients with nasal obstructions. • May cause headaches and will dry mucous membrane if oxygen therapy flow rates exceed $4\,L\,min^{-1}$. A bubble humidifier should be used in this situation. • Delivers unpredictable concentrations that vary with oxygen setting and with patient's ventilation pattern. (Bazuaye *et al.* 1992)

Table 5.6 *Continued.*

Name of oxygen delivery device/patient interface	Advantages	Disadvantages
Venturi mask 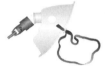	• Ideal for patients with type II and type I respiratory failure. • Venturi jets can be changed to deliver fixed oxygen concentrations (24–28–31–35–40–60%). • Delivers accurate oxygen concentrations irrespective of patients respiratory pattern and oxygen flow rate. • No rebreathing. (Khakhar *et al.* 2002)	• To meet the patients peak inspiratory flow requirements, the oxygen flow rate must be at least that indicated on valve. • Noisy, claustrophobic interferes with eating and drinking. • Mask cost higher than low flow medium concentration devices. • Variable output flow rates can be confusing. (Iooss *et al.* 1997)
Non-rebreathe masks	• Suitable for type I respiratory failure. • Allows delivery of approximately 95% oxygen concentration at flow rates of $12\,L\,min^{-1}$ (AHA 1997). • No rebreathing.	• Short-term use. • Uncomfortable for patients. • Ensure reservoir bag can expand freely and is not kinked. • Oxygen flow rate should be sufficient to keep the bag inflated.

Line drawings reproduced with permission from *Intersurgical®*.

procedures have also been called **non-invasive positive pressure ventilation** (NIPPV) despite the convention established by usage suggesting that the use of the term **non-invasive positive pressure ventilation** (NIPPV) should be limited to situations of type II respiratory failure (Antonelli *et al.* 1998).

Non-invasive ventilation

When NIV is prescribed, it should immediately initiate a pro-gramme to prepare the equipment necessary for full intubation should NIV fail. BTS (2002) produced guidelines on the prin-ciples of NIV including contraindications to its use. These include: raised intracranical pressure; impaired consciousness; pneumothorax (until a chest drain is sited); recent facial or upper airway surgery; facial abnormalities; vomiting. Patient refusal should also preclude the use of NIV.

NIV provides positive pressure to the patient's respiratory system. There are many machines that are used in the clinical situation to do this including BiPAP and CPAP. However the principles of operation are similar; it is not the aim of this book to provide extensive information on the principles of NIV but to illustrate the common features and provide a useful starting point for the novice practitioner in this area.

Benefits of NIV
- Reverses atelectasis.
- Improves oxygenation and reduces the work of breathing.
- Reduces cardiogenic pulmonary oedema.
- Improves cardiac function in some patients (Woodrow 2003).

Prior to the commencement of NIV a full and detailed patient assessment must be carried out. This should be completed by a multidisciplinary team and take into account the wishes of the patient and the family. A full explanation should be given to the patient and the patient given the chance to be involved con-structively in the selection process by experiencing the range of interfaces available.

Continuous positive airway pressure (CPAP)
The NIV equipment consists of a flow generator, oxygen analyser, pressure relief valve, humidifier, patient interface device and exit valve (see Fig. 5.2).

The flow generator, usually a bellows or a Venturi system, provides the driving system forcing the air to flow through the circuit. This air should be filtered by adding a bacterial filter

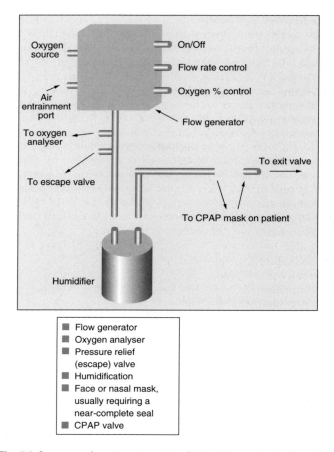

Fig. 5.2 Sequence of equipment used in CPAP. With permission from RCN Publishing (Woodrow 2003).

(Woodrow 2003). Supplemental oxygen is often entrained in the system and an oxygen analyser ensures that the amount of oxygen added into the circuit is adequate. The oxygen and flow rates should be calibrated at least once every eight hours. A pressure relief valve is included in the circuit to ensure that any obstruction in the system upstream of the exit valve does not result in large volumes of gas being delivered to the patient. The need for humidification in NIV circuits has already been discussed together with the caveats that apply to the control of temperature and the need for frequent checking.

The patient interface device should be tight fitting to minimise air leaks; however patients often find these masks painful and attempt to remove them at frequent intervals. By involving patients in the decision-making process there may be an improved compliance to the protocol and this risk may reduced.

The exit valve pressure is set such that most of the pressure generated by the patient on expiration will allow the egress of the inspired air. However at the end of expiration when expiratory pressure falls below the set value of the exit valve, the remaining air is 'trapped' within the circuit and airways thus providing additional airway support.

CPAP is a noisy and restrictive device; patients often find that it:

- reduces their mobility and independence;
- causes gastric distension;
- induces the formation of facial pressure sores, if a poorly fitted patient interface device is chosen;
- reduces lung compliance and increases cardiovascular instability (Woodrow 2003).

Invasive ventilation

Essentially this is the introduction of an airway adjunct such as endotracheal tube, which will allow the commencement of mechanical ventilation. The decision to undertake invasive ventilation is not made lightly and usually subsumes that the patient is rendered unconscious throughout the process. In an emergency situation it is usually only carried out in conditions of severe respiratory distress, although it is used routinely in some clinical areas, e.g. to maintain and provide anaesthesia during surgery. The work of breathing is undertaken by a machine, the 'ventilator' which will deliver a set volume of air (usually enriched with oxygen) and a set number of breaths per minute. The force that the air is delivered at is predetermined and the end expiratory pressure adjusted to ensure that the patient is receiving adequate ventilation.

LONG-TERM OXYGEN THERAPY (LTOT)

Long-term oxygen therapy is often prescribed for those patients with progressive lung disease, with the majority of those treated receiving oxygen therapy at home (Dunn & Chisholm 1998). The term LTOT generally refers to oxygen delivery periods greater than 15 hours per day including the time spent asleep (Smith 2004). LTOT has been proven to reduce polycythaemia (increased red blood cells due to the hypoxaemia) and pulmonary hypertension (Medical Research Council 1981). However more importantly the use of LTOT doubled the survival time of patients with chronic COPD in a clinical trial in 1981 (Medical Research Council 1981). This trial was ceased early due to the significant research findings and the promotion of LTOT for patients with chronic COPD commenced. If patients will comply and use LTOT for more than 15 hours a day, the positive effect upon life duration is enhanced (Plant & Elliott 2003).

LTOT is used to correct the chronic hypoxaemia associated with chronic lung diseases without causing carbon dioxide retention. The use of supplemental oxygen allows a greater concentration of oxygen within the arterial bloodstream, thus allowing a more normal level of cellular respiration. This then gives the patient more energy and a greater activity level than could be achieved without the use of LTOT. Other notable effects are reduced right-sided cardiac loading due to dilation of pulmonary arteries and a reduction in the stimulation of the carotid bodies responding to hypoxia and thus a reduced sensation of breathlessness.

Selection of patients to commence LTOT requires careful consideration and the optimisation of other therapy prior its commencement. These include smoking cessation therapy, maximisation of drug therapy and significant pulmonary rehabilitation (see Chapter 3). NICE guidelines (2004) provide advice on the selection of patients for the commencement of LTOT; these guidelines make it mandatory that the assessment of the patient should be overseen by a respiratory physician with suitable experience, and that the patient's condition should be stable with no recent exacerbations (Smith 2004).

Assessment of the patient in order to decide upon the concentration of oxygen therapy required is as follows (NICE 2004):

- Patients should be on maximum pharmacological therapy.
- Blood gases should be determined when the patient is stable, and measured on at least two occasions three weeks apart.
- $PaO_2 < 7.3\,kPa$ with or without CO_2 retention.
- $FEV_1 < 1.5\,L$ and $FVC < 2.0\,l$.
- PaO_2 between 7.3 and 8.0 kPa with evidence of pulmonary hypertension.

Patients have blood gases measured with supplemental oxygen, which initially commences at $1\,L\,min^{-1}$ for 20 minutes. Blood gases are rechecked and then assessed to indicate if hypoxaemia has been corrected with no increased carbon dioxide concentration. If the situation has not been corrected that oxygen level is increased to $2\,L\,min^{-1}$ and the process repeated. Once a level of oxygen therapy has been reached which corrects hypoxaemia without increasing carbon dioxide concentration, or the point is reached where the patient can tolerate no higher rate of oxygen flow, then these settings define the rate and concentration that the LTOT should be prescribed at.

Patients are re-assessed at least six-monthly to ensure hypoxaemia remains corrected and no other side effects of oxygen therapy are present.

At present hospital-based respiratory physicians within England cannot directly prescribed LTOT however this is not true in Scotland. In order to obtain oxygen therapy for these patients the hospital-based physician in England must contact the patient's GP and liaise with the GP to obtain the necessary prescription. However in 2005 this situation will alter and both GPs and hospital based physicians will be able to directly prescribe LTOT throughout the UK.

Once the decision to commence LTOT has been made, it will take up to four days for the company responsible for its set-up to contact the patient and organise the installation of an oxygen concentrator. The companies supplying the concentrator vary throughout the UK; the three main companies involved are BOC, DeVilbiss Healthcare and Oxygen Therapy Company Ltd.

An engineer will install the equipment and discuss its location and maintenance with patient and family. The provider has an obligation to service and maintain the equipment and provide 24-hour breakdown service.

Equipment used for LTOT

An oxygen concentrator is the most common means of delivering oxygen at home. It uses room air and removes nitrogen via filtration to produce oxygen. It runs off electricity and a back-up oxygen cylinder is always supplied in cases of electricity failure. The concentrator can deliver oxygen at a flow rate up to $4\,L\,min^{-1}$ and is delivered via oxygen tubing up to 50 m in length. It is efficient, cost-effective and a compact way of delivering oxygen, with significantly less storage space required than that taken up by several oxygen cylinders.

The choice of patient interface device is usually nasal cannulae, since these are tolerated quite well and have no significant issue of rebreathing associated with them. However the variable performance and fixed performance facemasks can be used with LTOT. The choice of patient interface device should be made after considering its compatibility with the equipment and the patient's preference. Patients should be given the contact names of the company that supplies their LTOT, the referring physician, GP and respiratory nurse/support team. Issues of smoking and the dangers of combustion should be clearly discussed with both the patient and their family.

Alternative methods of home oxygen provision include portable oxygen cylinders and liquid oxygen. Both these methods require a sizeable amount of storage space at the patient's home and this can be a limiting factor to the choice of oxygen delivery system recommended for home use.

The standard portable oxygen cylinder has a filling capacity of 230 L of compressed oxygen and weighs 2.3 kg (Esmond & Michalsons 2001). These cylinders will last 45 minutes if the flow rate is set at $4\,L\,min^{-1}$ or for a longer period at lower rates of flow. Larger cylinders are also available and those prescribed for home use will enable the smaller more portable cylinders to be re-filled when required.

SUMMARY

❏ Oxygen therapy is widely used in all clinical care situations.
❏ Oxygen therapy is a medication and should be prescribed for each individual patient except in situations of life threatening emergencies.
❏ The assessment of patients before they commence or cease oxygen therapy is essential.
❏ Accurate documentation of all vital observations and clinical information should be carried out.
❏ Choice of oxygen delivery system depends upon many factors, patient choice and comfort being not the least important.
❏ Long-term and/or high flow oxygen therapy should be humidified.
❏ Long-term oxygen therapy should be considered in cases of severe COPD.
❏ The use of non-invasive and invasive ventilation should be considered in cases of severe respiratory failure, with designated and appropriately qualified personnel appointed to provide care and support for the patient and family.

REFERENCES

Ahern J, Philpot P (2002) Assessing acutely ill patients on general wards. *Nursing Standard* **16** (47): 54–57.

American Heart Association (1997) *Pediatric advanced life support*. Dallas, TX, AHA.

Antonelli M, Conti G, Rocco M *et al.* (1998) A comparison of non-invasive positive pressure ventilation and conventional mechanical ventilation in patients with acute respiratory failure. *New England Journal of Medicine* **397** (7): 429–435.

Ashurst S (1995) Oxygen therapy. *British Journal of Nursing* **4** (9): 508–515.

Bateman NT, Leech RM (1998) ABC of oxygen: acute oxygen therapy. *British Medical Journal* **317**: 798–801.

Bazuaye EA, Stone TN, Corris PA, Gibson GJ (1992) Variability of inspired oxygen concentration with nasal cannulas. *Thorax* **47** (12): 1086.

Bell C (1995) Is this what the doctor ordered? Accuracy of oxygen therapy prescribed and delivered in hospital. *Professional Nurse* **10** (5): 297–300.

Bennett C (2002) Respiratory care. In: Workman B, Bennett C (2002) *Key nursing skills.* Whurr, London.

Bennett C (2003) Nursing the breathless patient. *Nursing Standard* **17** (17): 45–51.

Bourke SJ (2003) *Lecture notes on respiratory medicine*, 6th edn. Blackwell Publishing, Oxford.

British Thoracic Society (2002) Non invasive ventilation in acute respiratory failure. *Thorax* **57** (3): 192–211.

Clutton-Brock T (1997) The assessment and monitoring of respiratory function. In: Goldhill D, Withington P (eds) *Textbook of intensive care.* Chapman & Hall, London.

Coombs M (2001) Making sense of arterial blood gases. *Nursing Times* **97** (27): 36–38.

Dunn L, Chisholm H (1998) Oxygen therapy. *Nursing Standard* **13** (7): 57–64.

Esmond G, Mikelsons C (2001) Oxygen therapy. In: Esmond G (ed.) *Respiratory nursing.* Baillière Tindall, Edinburgh.

Fell H, Boehm M (1998) Easing the discomfort of oxygen therapy. *Nursing Times* **94** (38): 56–58.

Guyton A, Hall J (2000) *Textbook of medical physiology*, 10th edn. WB Saunders, Philadelphia.

Iooss P, Sellal KO, Legoff S, Grimandi G (1997) Evaluation study of seven Venturi face mask. *Pharmacie Hospitaliere Francaise* Spec Issue 3–5.

Jeffrey AA, Warren PM (1992) Should we judge a mask by its cover? *Thorax* **47** (7): 543–546.

Jevon P, Ewens B (2001) Assessment of a breathless patient. *Nursing Standard* **15** (16): 48–53.

Khakhar M, Heah T, Al-Shaikh B (2002) Oxygen delivery systems for the spontaneously breathing patient. *CPD Anaesthesia* **4** (1): 27–30.

Lifecare (2000) *Product information.* Lifecare Hospital Supplies, Market Harborough.

Medical Research Council (1981) Long term domiciliary oxygen therapy in chronic hypoxic cor pulmonale complicating chronic bronchitis and emphysema. *Lancet* **1** (8222): 681–686.

NICE (2004) COPD guidelines. *Thorax* **59** (Suppl. 1).

Penney D, LePoidevin R, Harmer M (2000) Blocked oxygen tubing. *Anaesthesia* **55** (7): 724–725.

Pilkington F (2004) Humidification for oxygen therapy in non-ventilated patients. *British Journal of Nursing* **13** (2): 111–115.

Plant P, Elliott M (2003) Chronic obstructive pulmonary disease: management of ventilatory failure in COPD. *Thorax* **58**: 537–542.

Sasaki H, Yamakage M, Iwasaki S *et al.* (2003) Design of oxygen delivery systems influences both effectiveness to comfort in adult volunteers. *Canadian Journal of Anaesthesia.* **50** (10): 1052–1055.

Sheppard M, Davis S (2000) Practical procedures for nurses – oxygen therapy: 1. *Nursing Times* **96** (29): 43–44.

Simmons P, Simmons M (2004) Informed nursing practice: the administration of oxygen to patients with COPD. *Medsurgical Nursing* **13** (2): 82–86.

Smith GB, Poplett N (2002) Knowledge of aspects of acute care in trainee doctors. *Postgraduate Medical Journal* **78** (920): 335–338.

Smith T (2004) Oxygen therapy for older people. *Nursing Older People* **16** (5): 22–28.

Torrance C, Elley K (1997) Respiration, technique and observation 1. *Nursing Times* **93** (43): Suppl. 1–2.

Vines DL, Shelledy DC, Peters J (2000) Current respiratory care. Part 1: Oxygen therapy, oximetry, bronchial hygiene – among many devices and methods, how to choose those that meet therapeutic goals. *Journal of Critical Illness* **15** (9): 507–515.

Woodcock A, Partridge M (1996) *Respiratory handbook.* Boehringer, Ingelheim.

Woodrow P (2003) Using non-invasive ventilation in acute wards: Part 1. *Nursing Standard* **17** (18) 1: 39–44.

Lung Cancer and Thoracic Surgical Intervention

Lung cancer has increased in prevalence and incidence since the early 20th century (Finkelmeier 2000). It has now reached the status of being one of the most common malignant diseases and a major problem throughout the world, in the USA an estimated 171 500 new cases of lung cancer are diagnosed each year (Landis *et al.* 1998), and in the UK it kills *circa* 38 000 people each year (Bourke 2003).

Lung cancer develops most frequently in late middle age or within the older population; it occurs more often in men than in women, but the incidence in women is increasing (Finkelmeier 2000). The ratio of men to women was formally 8 : 1; it is now less than 2 : 1 (Shields 1994).

This chapter aims to:
- Outline the management of patients with lung cancer and their families. Discuss the management and treatment of: pleural effusions; pneumothorax and empyema.
- Discuss the management of patients with chest drains *in situ*.
- Outline the common thoracic surgical procedures used to obtain a diagnosis or give treatment for thoracic conditions.

LUNG CANCER

Risk factors in the development of lung cancer are manifold and include race and ethnicity (Finkelmeier 2000). However the major risk taking activity that increases the probability of developing lung cancer is cigarette tobacco smoking. It is believed to be responsible for 80% of lung cancer cases (Baldini & Strauss 1997).

The duration of cigarette smoking, the number of cigarettes smoked per day and the amount of nicotine and tar in the cigarettes smoked are all interrelated and 'quantify' the risk of developing lung cancer. Benfield & Russell (1996) provided evidence that a cohort of heavy smokers have 25 times as many cases of lung cancers as a similar size population of non-smokers. Heavy smoking is defined in the UK in terms of pack years smoked (see Chapter 3). Cessation of smoking will reduce the risk of developing lung cancer; however those who have smoked will throughout their lifetime still have a higher risk of developing lung cancer than those who have never smoked (Mulshine & Tockman 1992).

Passive smoking is also known as a cause of lung cancer; it is estimated that a women who has never smoked will have a 24% greater chance of developing lung cancer if she lives with a partner who smokes (Bourke 2003).

Other carcinogens that can increase the predisposition for the development of lung cancer are asbestos, radioactive material, arsenic, nickel and numerous organic chemicals (Shields 1994).

Pathology of lung cancer

Bronchogenic carcinoma is cancer which arises from the epithelial lining of the bronchi; it is the most common form of lung cancer and accounts for approximately 90% of cases (Finkelmeier 2000). This type of cancer is then further subdivided as illustrated in Figure 6.1.

Adenocarcinoma comprises 50% of lung tumours (D'Amico & Sabiston 1995). It is increasing in incidence and occurs more commonly in women than in men. It is the lung cancer most likely to develop in non-smokers (Sridhar & Raub 1992). The survival rate is greater for this type of lung cancer than in any other.

Squamous carcinoma comprises 30–35% of lung cancer, occurring most frequently in people with a long smoking history.

Small cell carcinoma accounts for 20–25% of lung cancer; most people with this cancer have a smoking history. It is a highly malignant and is characterised by a rapid tumour doubling time, early and widespread dissemination and relatively short patient survival. Due to its rapid spread, surgical resection is uncommon.

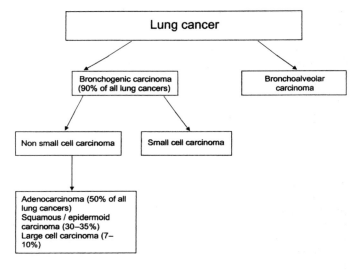

Fig. 6.1 Pathology of lung cancer.

Bronchoalveolar carcinoma originates in the lung parenchyma. It spreads along the alveolar walls. It is also known as alveolar carcinoma, bronchioalveolar carcinoma and bronchiolar carcinoma.

Lung tumours can disseminate throughout the body by three main routes: firstly by direct extension, secondly spread by the lymphatic system, and finally by haematologic spread. The most common sites of lung cancer metastasis are listed in Table 6.1.

Staging of lung cancer

This is vital in order to: classify the extent of the disease; direct the therapy required; and provide more accurate prognostic information. Standard nomenclature for pathologic classification exists and has been developed since 1978. The most recent and universal system adopted is based on the International

Table 6.1 Sites of lung tumour spread.

Common sites of lung cancer metastasis
Contralateral lung
Brain
Cervical nodes
Liver
Bone
Adrenals
Skin

Staging System, which consists of a three-letter code. The first letter is 'T' which categorises tumour size, the second 'N' the presence and extent of nodule involvement and the third 'M' the presence of direct metastasis (Mountain 1997). The staging is also determined by the position of the tumour and not just size. Tumours can be accurately staged in 80% of cases using CT.

Clinical manifestations

It has been found that 90–95% of patients with lung cancer are symptomatic at the time of diagnosis (Shields 1994). The clinical signs and symptoms depend on size and location of the tumour, extent of spread to adjacent or distant structures and occurrence of associated hormonal syndromes. Cough occurs in most patients and many have persistent upper respiratory tract infections or pneumonia due to bronchial obstruction. Other pulmonary manifestations include haemoptysis, dyspnoea, wheezing and lung abscess (Maddaus & Ginsberg 1995). Non-specific symptoms associated with lung cancer include weight loss, anorexia and malaise.

Investigations

Patients will experience a number of investigations; however the most frequent will be a simple chest X-ray. A large range of abnormalities may become apparent which are suggestive of cancer.

Sputum cytology will be positive in 40% of lung cancers, while bronchoscopy will allow the direct visualisation of some central tumours.

Other investigations that might be carried out include percutaneous needle biopsy of lesions under radiological guidance and even CT and MRI scanning. Occasionally needle-guided biopsies are inconclusive or technically difficult; in these cases video-assisted thoracic surgery, mediastinoscopy; and mini-thoracotomy are options to obtain tissue for diagnoses.

TREATMENT OF LUNG CANCER

Survival prognosis of patients diagnosed with lung cancer is poor. Some 10–13% of patients will survive 5 years after diagnosis. For non-small cell lung cancer the treatment of choice is surgical resection of the tumour and surrounding lymphatic tissue. For non-small cell cancer and in early stage small cell cancer surgical resection has been demonstrated to increase five-year survival rates to as much as 50–70% (Sheppard *et al.* 1991). The selection of the specific operative procedure depends upon: the location and size of the tumour; its spread to lymph nodes; involvement of extra-pulmonary structures; and the patient's age and medical condition. Figure 6.2 outlines the British Thoracic Society (2003b) recommendations that should be borne in mind whenever the suitability for surgery of patients with lung cancer is being considered.

Lobectomy (removal of an entire lobe) is generally considered the minimum definitive pulmonary resection; removal of two lobes (bi-lobectomy) or an entire lung (pneumonectomy) may be necessary if the tumour is centrally located or involves more than one lobe. The respiratory function that the patient is likely to be left with in each of these cases, is a significant factor that is taken into consideration during the selection of patients for surgery.

Although surgical treatment is the most effective therapy for non-small cell lung cancer, only 30–40% of patients are suitable for curative resection (Carney 1998). Surgical resection is usually only one component in the treatment approach of lung

Summary of recommendations

PART I: FITNESS FOR SURGERY
Age
1. Perioperative morbidity increases with advancing age. Elderly patients undergoing lung resection are more likely to require intensive perioperative support. Preoperatively, a careful assessment of co-morbidity needs to be made.
2. Surgery for clinically stage I and II disease can be as effective in patients over 70 years as in younger patients. Such patients should be considered for surgical treatment regardless of age.
3. Age over 80 alone is not a contraindication to lobectomy or wedge resection for clinically stage I disease.
4. Pneumonectomy is associated with a higher mortality risk in the elderly. Age should be a factor in deciding suitability for pneumonectomy.

Pulmonary function
1. There should be formal liaison in borderline cases between the referring chest physician and the thoracic surgical team.
2. No further respiratory function tests are required for a lobectomy if the post-bronchodilator FEV_1 is >1.5 litres and for a pneumonectomy if the post-bronchodilator FEV_1 is >2.0 litres, provided that there is no evidence of interstitial lung disease or unexpected disability due to shortness of breath.

STEP 1
3. All patients not clearly operable on the basis of spirometry should have: (a) full pulmonary function tests including estimation of transfer factor (T_{Lco}); (b) measurement of oxygen saturation on air at rest; and (c) a quantitative isotope perfusion scan if a pneumonectomy is being considered.
4. These data should be used to calculate estimated postoperative FEV_1 expressed as % predicted and the estimated postoperative T_{lco} expressed as % predicted, using either the lung scan for pneumonectomy or an anatomical equation for lobectomy, taking account of whether the segments to be removed are ventilated or obstructed.

STEP 2
5. (a) Estimated postoperative FEV_1 >40% predicted and estimated postoperative T_{Lco} >40% predicted and oxygen saturation (Sao_2) >90% on air: average risk.
   (b) Estimated postoperative FEV_1 <40% predicted and estimated postoperative T_{Lco} <40% predicted: high risk.
   (c) All other combinations: consider exercise testing.
6. Patients for whom the risk of resection is still unclear after step 2 tests should be referred for exercise testing.

STEP 3
7. (a) A best distance on two shuttle walk tests of <25 shuttles (250 m) or desaturation during the test of more than 4% Sao_2 indicates a patient is a high risk for surgery.

Fig. 6.2 BTS recommendations for selection of patients for surgery. With permission, BMJ Publishing Group (BTS 2001).

(b) Other patients should be referred for a formal cardiopulmonary exercise test. For cardiopulmonary exercise testing peak oxygen consumption ($\dot{V}O_2$peak) of more than 15 mL/kg/min indicates that a patient is an average risk for surgery.

(c) A $\dot{V}O_2$peak of <15 ml/kg/min indicates that a patient is high risk for surgery.

HIGH RISK PATIENTS

8. The management of these patients should be considered at a formal multidisciplinary meeting between a chest physician, surgeon, and an oncologist.

9. Such patients could be considered for a more limited resection; radiotherapy/chemotherapy.

Cardiovascular fitness

1. All patients for lung resection should have a preoperative ECG.
2. All patients with an audible cardiac murmur should have an echocardiogram.
3. Patients who have had a myocardial infarction should normally not be operated on for lung resection within 6 weeks.
4. Any patient who has had a myocardial infarction within 6 months and is being assessed for thoracic surgery should have a cardiology opinion.
5. Patients who have had coronary artery bypass surgery should not be precluded from having lung resection. They should be assessed as for other patients with possible cardiac risk factors.
6. The guidelines from the American College of Cardiology and the American Heart Association should be used as a basis for assessing the perioperative cardiovascular risk of patients undergoing lung resection.

MAJOR RISK

(a) These patients should have a formal cardiological assessment and their management discussed at a multidisciplinary meeting.

(b) Patients found to have significant lesions on coronary angiography should be considered for coronary artery bypass surgery before lung resection.

INTERMEDIATE RISK

(a) Patients in this group with reasonable functional capacity (able comfortably to walk up one flight of stairs) should not normally be regarded as at greater than average risk for postoperative complications. They do not need further cardiac testing.

(b) Patients with poor functional capacity and those in whom there is doubt about the degree of severity of their angina pectoris or who report breathlessness which may be due to cardiac disease should have an ECG monitored exercise test and echocardiogram and the results should be discussed with a cardiologist.

MINOR RISK

Patients in this group with one risk factor should not normally be considered to be at greater than average risk for postoperative complication.

7. Particular care should be taken in patients presenting with more than one cardiovascular risk factor.

Fig. 6.2 *Continued.*

8. All patients with a history of previous stroke, transient ischaemic attacks, or carotid bruits should be assessed by carotid Doppler studies. Patients with evidence of significant stenoses (for example, over 70%) should be assessed by a vascular surgeon or consultant in stroke medicine preoperatively and their management discussed with the thoracic surgeon.

Weight loss, performance status and nutrition
1. Patients presenting with a preoperative weight loss of 10% or more and/or a performance status of WHO 2 or worse are highly likely to have advanced disease and to require particularly careful staging assessment, together with a search for evidence of co-morbidity.
2. Routine preoperative assessment should include a simple measure of nutritional status such as the body mass index, together with a serum albumin measurement. Low values should be accepted as conveying an increased risk of postoperative complications.

Multiple risk factors
1. Patients anatomically suitable for resection but with more than one adverse medical factor should have their management discussed formally at a multidisciplinary meeting between a chest physician, a surgeon and an oncologist.

PART II: OPERABILITY
Diagnosis and staging
1. All patients being considered for surgery should have a plain chest radiograph and a computed tomographic (CT) scan of the thorax including the liver and adrenal glands.
2. Confirmatory diagnostic percutaneous needle biopsy in patients presenting with peripheral lesions is not mandatory in patients who are otherwise fit, particularly if there are previous chest radiographs showing no evidence of a lesion.
3. Patients with mediastinal nodes greater than 1 cm in short axis diameter on the CT scan should undergo biopsy by staging mediastinoscopy, anterior mediastinotomy, or needle biopsy as appropriate.

Operability and adjuvant therapy
1. The proportion of patients found to be inoperable at operation should be 5–10%.
2. Patients with stage I (cT1N0 and cT2N0) and stage II (cT1N1, cT2N1 and cT3N0) tumours should be considered operable.
3. Patients with stage I tumours have a high chance and those with stage II tumours a reasonable chance of being cured by surgery alone.
4. Patients known preoperatively to have stage IIIA (cT3N1 and cT1–3N2) tumours have a low chance of being cured by surgery alone but might be considered operable in the context of a trial of surgery and adjuvant chemotherapy.
5. Participation in prospective trials of multimodality treatment for locally advanced disease is strongly recommended.

Fig. 6.2 *Continued.*

6. Some small individual studies indicate a place for surgery in T4N0 and T4N1 tumours within stage IIIB, few long term data are available. Generally, stage IIIB tumours with node involvement and stage IV tumours should be considered inoperable.
7. There is no place for postoperative radiotherapy following complete primary tumour resection.

Operations available
1. Sublobar resection is a useful option in patients with impaired pulmonary reserve, but there is a higher local recurrence rate than with lobectomy and long term survival is decreased by 5–10%.
2. Mortality following resection should not be in excess of 4% for lobectomy and 8% for pneumonectomy.
3. Bronchoplastic resection may be appropriate in patients with impaired pulmonary reserve and in selected patients with advanced endobronchial lesions.
4. Carinal resection is a technically demanding procedure with significant potential for major postoperative problems and an increased risk of local recurrence. Consideration should be given to concentrating such surgery in a few centres.
5. The use of video-assisted thoracic surgery (VATS) for the resection of bronchogenic carcinoma is rare and limited data are available. It causes less postoperative pain than open surgery and appears to give similar long term results.
6. Systematic lymph node dissection at the time of lung resection is essential to achieve accurate staging.
7. The therapeutic value of radical lymphadenectomy is uncertain.

Locally advanced disease
1. The management of individual patients with locally advanced disease should be discussed at multidisciplinary meetings involving physicians, surgeons, and oncologists.
2. The results or surgery for locally invasive non-small cell lung cancer (NSCLC) are good when the lateral chest wall is involved.
3. Highly selected patients with vertebral column involvement or superior sulcus tumours may be suitable for radical surgery, possibly in combination with other treatments.
4. There is no case for surgery in these groups when mediastinal lymph nodes are involved.

Small cell lung cancer
1. Surgery is appropriate treatment for stage I small cell lung cancer (SCLC).
2. The incidence of subclinical metastatic disease is much higher in SCLC than in NSCLC and all patients being considered for surgery should be staged by CT scanning and mediastinoscopy and screened by scanning of bones and brain and iliac crest bone marrow sampling.
3. Patients with small peripheral nodules should not be denied consideration for surgery on the basis of a needle biopsy showing SCLC.

Fig. 6.2 *Continued.*

cancer; other modalities of treatment include radiation therapy and chemotherapy, which are the focus of many current studies.

Preoperative patient care of those with lung cancer

This includes both physical and psychological preparation (Finkelmeier 2000). Preoperative evaluation by both the medical and nursing profession should complement each other. It is aimed at providing baseline information that will allow greater interpretation of the postoperative findings. The preoperative period will allow the nurse to establish relationships with both the family and the patient, and provides the opportunity for the team of health professionals to give the essential information concerning the surgical procedure and postoperative care that the patient will undergo.

A full detailed patient examination and assessment will be undertaken; this may be carried out by nurse practitioners and will be written in both medical and nursing notes of the patient. Lung cancer patients will often have other co-morbidities associated with them. These are important factors that are often of paramount concern in arriving at the decision to perform surgery or not. Common co-morbidities include chronic obstructive pulmonary disease, coronary artery disease, hypertension and diabetes mellitus.

Preoperative instruction will include: outlining the type of care that the patient will experience; likely length of stay in hospital; the overall programmed postoperative recovery and any information that the patient will need to increase their recovery rate post-surgery. The type of procedure that the patient is to experience should be clearly explained to the patient in a language and manner that is suitable for their comprehension. This increases the patient's understanding of the procedure and reduces the chance of the patient having a different expectation to that which the reality of the experience makes possible (Clark & Ihde 1998).

Many patients will receive and undergo surgery very soon after their lung cancer has been diagnosed, thus patients are often very anxious and may not have had sufficient time to contact their GP or other health professionals to allay their fears.

This anxiety needs special consideration by all health professionals when explaining to the patient about their forthcoming operation. Clear expectations should be given to the patient concerning their immediate postoperative care and this should include: pain management; the importance of post-surgery ambulation; coughing techniques and deep breathing techniques that are important to help mobilise secretions and prevent atelectasis.

Pain management should be addressed in preoperative information given to patients to aid in their postoperative recovery. In most cases a thoracic epidural or paravertebral block will be sited to allow pain relief to be given to the patient in the first few days post-surgery. Other methods of pain relief include patient-controlled intravenous analgesia or intermittent dosing of opioid analgesia.

During the several (usually two, rarely three) days after surgery, the higher levels of analgesia are continued to allow deep breathing and coughing. Oral analgesia is not usually used in the immediate postoperative days since it requires the patient to be sufficiently well enough before they can tolerate oral fluids. Therefore the alternative methods of patient pain relief are continued. As soon as possible oral analgesia is implemented (typically codeine, paracetamol and anti-inflammatories) and the initial methods of pain relief discontinued.

Postoperative management of thoracic surgical patients

Immediately following the procedure the patient will be transferred either into the recovery area, or if extensive surgery and related patient co-morbidities are present they may be transferred to intensive care/high care areas. The principles of immediate postoperative management are the same however, and centre around maintaining the patient's cardiovascular and respiratory systems in order to promote homeostasis.

It is crucial that the nurse caring for the patient is fully informed as to the procedure undertaken in theatre, what anaesthesia was used and any significant intraoperative findings or complications, amount of intraoperative fluids transfused and any current medication and fluids in progress.

Evidence also shows that patients with a chest drain should be cared for by nurses who are not only fully familiar with the relevant guidelines, but are also frequently required to exercise the necessary skills when caring for patients with chest drains (BTS 2003a).

The nurse must re-establish or continue the monitoring that is mandated for the patient. This will involve ECG monitoring, peripheral pulse oximetry and sometimes arterial blood gas monitoring. If the patient is being ventilated, to minimise the risk of hypoxaemia, it must be ensured that the correct and appropriate ventilation is being delivered. Vital signs are monitored to assess the patient's haemodynamic stability and as part of an overall assessment of the patient's condition. All catheters should be checked for patency and intravenous fluid infusion assessed to assure appropriate fluid delivery rates. Chest drain management should be carried out (see below). Breath sounds should be auscultated at suitable intervals for the patient. This is often undertaken by the multidisciplinary team and occurs frequently throughout the patient's treatment, typically on insertion of the drain, administration of physiotherapy and removal of the drain.

Supplemental oxygen delivery is usually required and the duration of this can be several days. In these cases supplemental oxygen should always be humidified.

The patient condition will dictate the frequency of vital sign observation and this is usually guided by the local policies in each thoracic surgical unit.

Pain management should be addressed and pain assessment scales should be used to provide appropriate pain relief to the patient.

As the patient improves, their mobility and respiratory function should increase and there should be a clear plan for their discharge home. Discharge should consider the full integration of the primary care team who will continue to support the patient and their family. Many thoracic surgical units will have nurse specialists in lung cancer who will establish a link with the patient and provide clinical contact for them and their families. Regular review and follow-up in 'Outpatients' clinics are mandatory. Since the survival rate for those with lung cancer is quite low, it is highly likely that those patients will be reviewed and receive palliative care later in their life. This is an important prognostic factor that should be discussed with patients.

Palliative care

The focus of palliative care is to maximise patient's functioning and quality of life. Palliative care is provided by experienced health care professionals who are able to take over the expert care required for symptom management such as pain relief, malaise, fatigue and anorexia. It is important to establish a link with the palliative care team early in the patient's diagnosis so that the therapeutic relationships can be established. In some instances this may be via the lung cancer specialist; however local policies and guidelines should be able to provide specific advice concerning this area.

PNEUMOTHORAX

This is defined as air in the pleural space, i.e. air between the lung and chest wall (Light 1995).

Pneumothoraces are either primary or secondary in origin. Primary pneumothoraces occur in otherwise healthy individuals; it is a significant global problem occurring in 18–28 per 100 000 men each year and in 1.2–6 per 100 000 women per year (Melton *et al.* 1979, Benese *et al.* 1987). Patients with primary pneumothorax show symptoms that include breathlessness and a reduced exercise tolerance. Small primary pneumothoraces (less than 2 cm diameter BTS 2003a) often resolve spontaneously, but even so they do deserve close monitoring of the patient. The patient with a small primary pneumothorax will often delay seeking medical treatment for two or more days (BTS 2003a), but upon presentation the patient may have abnormal arterial blood gas analysis but fairly normal lung function results.

Pneumothoraces which are greater than 2 cm will require intervention, either simple aspiration (thoracocentesis), insertion of a chest drain and/or referral to a chest physician.

Secondary pneumothoraces arise in response to lung cancer metastases, cystic fibrosis, asthma, COPD, and lung infections, and require more than observation (BTS 2003a). These symptoms tend to be more severe than those with primary pneumothoraces, the patients complaining of breathlessness greater in severity than would be expected due to the size of the pneumothorax. They require the hospital admission of the patient and commencement of supplemental oxygen, insertion of a chest drain and direct care under the supervision of a chest or thoracic surgeon.

In summary the BTS advocate conservative or minimalistic approaches to resolution of a pneumothorax. However if two or more pneumothoraces have occurred then referral should be made to a thoracic surgeon for video-assisted thoracoscopic (VATS) and partial pleurectomy.

EMPYEMA

This is pleural infection, characterised by pus within the pleural space (Selby 2002). The increased use of antibiotics has seen a reduction in empyema incidence, however there has been an increase in anaerobic infections and Gram-negative organisms. Treatment comprises insertion of a chest tube and in some cases the intervention of video-assisted thoracoscopic (VATS) pleural debridement (Wait *et al.* 1997).

Clinical features of empyema

These include fever, systemic upset and pleural discomfort. If a pneumonia is present this can confound the clinical picture and provide problems with detection of pleural fluid. The lack of response to antibiotic therapy should prompt further investigation into the clinical condition of the patient and considerations of the existence of empyema.

Management of empyema

A large-bore intercostal drainage tube should be inserted, and its management carefully monitored. Antibiotic therapy should also be given, and the choice of the antibiotic should be based upon the results of a culture response. A broad-spectrum antibiotic could be prescribed to control any anaerobic organisms (Selby 2002).

Thoracic surgery is frequently required to remove the pleural thickening that can occur after the development of an empyema. If left the pleural thickening can calcify and restrict the complete re-expansion of the affected lung. Thoracotomy, rib resection and decortication are frequently performed.

CHEST DRAINS

Chest drains are inserted in many different clinical settings, the principles of insertion and management are discussed below.

The indications for the insertion of a chest drain are numerous however the most common reasons are illustrated in Table 6.2. These are taken from the British Thoracic Society (2003b) guidelines for the insertion of a chest drain.

All the equipment required to insert the drain should be available before commencing the procedure. If the patient is able to provide it, the consent of the patient should be obtained. Written information should always be provided. However in situations of life-saving intervention when the patient is unable to give consent, then the procedure should be carried out and the patient fully informed of the procedure as soon as possible thereafter.

Table 6.2 Indications for insertion of a chest drain.

Pneumothorax
  In any ventilated patient.
  Tension pneumothorax after initial needle relief.
  Persistent or recurrent pneumothorax after simple aspiration.
  Large secondary spontaneous pneumothorax in patients over 50 years.
Malignant pleural effusion.
Empyema and complicated parapneumonic pleural effusion.
Traumatic haemopneumothorax.
Postoperative – for example, thoracotomy, oesophagectomy, cardiac surgery.

Reproduced from BTS guidelines for the insertion of a chest drain (2003) *Thorax* **58** (Suppl. II): ii53–ii59. With permission from BMJ Publishing Group.

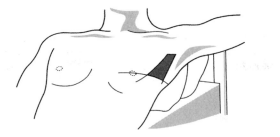

Fig. 6.3 Insertion site of chest drains. With permission from BMJ Publishing Group (BTS 2003b).

The insertion of a chest drain is a highly painful procedure; 50% of patients experience pain levels of 9–10 on a scale of 10 (Luketich *et al.* 1998) and thus appropriate pain relief should be administered. This should ideally be in the form of pre-medication (before the event) and then followed up by post chest drain insertion analgesia.

Patients are positioned in bed either upright leaning over an adjacent table with a pillow or on their bed with the arm on the side of the lesion up behind their head to expose the axillary area (see Fig. 6.3).

The 'drain' chosen should reflect its main aim; previously large-bore tubes were used since it was felt that these were not as prone to occlusion as smaller bore tubes (BTS 2003b). However it is now common practice to use small-bore tubes since these are more comfortable for the patient and thus better tolerated; they do not appear to occlude any more frequently than the larger bore tubes, but this evidence is anecdotal and needs further investigation. Acute haemothorax does merit the use of large-bore chest drains (28–30 F minimum); this is to aid in the drainage from the thoracic cavity and assessment of continuing blood loss.

The insertion of a chest drain should be via an aseptic technique and performed without substantial force (BTS 2003b). This is not a nursing procedure, so will not be outlined further in this chapter. However the nurse's role is vital to care for the patient and provide comfort and reassurance.

Once the chest drain is inserted, it should be securely fixed so as to avoid its accidental removal. It should not be secured by the use of large amounts of tape and padding since this would restrict the natural movement of the patient's chest wall. Excessive tape and padding use can obscure accidental disconnection of the chest drain. The chest drain should be securely anchored in place by sutures (see BTS 2003b for further information).

Once inserted and securely anchored the chest drain is attached to a drainage system. The management of the chest drain is of particular relevance to the nurse. Chest drains should be connected to a single flow drainage system, for example an under water seal bottle or flutter valve.

The closed underwater seal bottle is the most popular system. A tube is placed under water to an approximate depth of 3 cm, with a side vent which will allow escape of air, or the tube may be connected to a suction pump. The use of an underwater seal bottle will ensure that air bubbles can be seen as the lung re-expands in cases of pneumothorax or allow a visible estimation to be made of the fluid evacuation rate in empyemas, pleural effusions or haemothorax. The fluid in the bottle should swing upon inspiration and expiration of the patient and this allows the assessment of the patency of the chest drain. If an underwater seal system is used this ensures minimum problems for inpatient management of the patient. However there is the difficulty of patient mobilisation, and the additional risks of knocking over the bottle. Chest tubes should be managed on specialist wards by staff who are trained in chest drain management and this practice is the one recommended by the British Thoracic Society (BTS). See Fig. 6.4 outlining basic properties of an underwater chest drain.

Once inserted a chest X-ray should be performed to assess the position of the tube and exclude any complications that can occur upon the insertion of chest drains.

The use of suction has been recommended in cases of non-resolving pneumothorax or following chemical pleurodesis (Harris and Graham 1991, BTS 2003b). If suction is required this

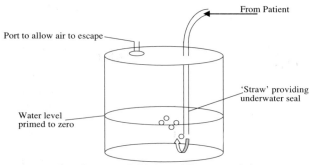

Port to allow air to escape

From Patient

'Straw' providing underwater seal

Water level primed to zero

An underwater sealed drain providing one way drainage.

Fig. 6.4 Underwater chest drain.

may be performed via the underwater seal at a level of negative pressure equivalent to 10–20 cm of water. A wall suction adaptor may also be used, but under no circumstances must chest drains be connected directly to the high negative pressure available from wall suction.

Chest drains must be observed and there should be appropriate documentation of drainage and any possible complications. This documentation should also be used to indicate what type of analgesics are required by the patient in order to aid in mobilisation. The duration of chest tube drainage should be recorded; all this information will aid in the decision as to when to remove the chest drain. These are all important 'landmark' points that should be followed in the management of chest drains and are the audit points suggested by the BTS.

Clamping of chest drains

There are some general principles that should be followed to aid in the decision as to whether to clamp a chest drain or not. These are clearly outlined in the BTS guidelines for the insertion of chest drains (2003b). Expert opinion suggests that:

- A bubbling chest drain should never be clamped.
- Drainage of a large pleural effusion should be controlled to ensure no more than 500 mL per hour of drainage is obtained.
- In cases of pneumothorax clamping of chest tubes should usually be avoided.
- If a chest tube is clamped this should be under suitable direct care of an appropriate chest physician or thoracic surgeon and cared for upon a ward staffed by nurses with suitable experience.
- If the patient develops breathlessness the drain should be immediately unclamped and medical advice sought.

Removal of the chest drain should be either while the patient performs the Valsalva manoeuvre or during expiration. It requires two health care professionals to remove the drain: one to remove the chest drain and the other to tie the suture in place upon its removal to effect the closure of the chest drain insertion site. Clamping of the drain prior to its removal is usually not required (BTS 2003b). In the case of a pneumothorax the drain should not usually be removed until bubbling from the chest drain has ceased; a chest X-ray should demonstrate lung re-inflation has occurred (Treasure and Murphy 1989).

SUMMARY
This chapter has considered the management of patients with:

❑ Lung cancer.
❑ Pneumothorax.
❑ Empyema.
❑ Chest drains.

It has explored the use of a multiprofessional team in the management of lung cancer and considered briefly the role of palliative care.

REFERENCES
Baldini EH, Strauss GM (1997) Women and lung cancer: waiting to exhale. *Chest* **112** (Suppl. 4): 229S.
Benese L, Wiman LG, Hedenstierna G (1987) Onset of symptoms in spontaneous pneumothorax: correlations to physical activity. *European Journal of Respiratory Disease* **71**: 181–186.

Benfield JR, Russell LA (1996) Lung carcinomas. In: Baue AE, Geha AS, Hammond GL *et al.* (eds) *Glenn's thoracic and cardiovascular surgery*, 6th edn. Appleton & Lange, Stamford.

Bourke SJ (2003) *Respiratory medicine*, 6th edn. Blackwell Publishing, Oxford.

BTS (2003a) BTS Guidelines for the management of pleural disease. *Thorax* **58** (Suppl. I): ii1–iii59.

BTS (2003b) BTS Guidelines for the insertion of a chest drain. *Thorax* **58** (Suppl. II): ii53–ii59.

Carney DN (1998) New agents in the management of advanced non-small cell lung cancer. *Seminal Oncology* **25**: 83.

Clark R, Ihde DC (1998) Small cell lung cancer: treatment progress and prospects. *Oncology* **12**: 647.

D'Amico TA, Sabiston DC (1995) Carcinoma of the lung. In: Sabiston DC, Spencer FC (eds) *Surgery of the chest*, 6th edn. WB Saunders, Philadelphia.

Finkelmeier BA (2000) *Cardiothoracic surgical nursing*, 2nd edn. Lippincott, Philadelphia.

Harris DR, Graham TR (1991) Management of intercostal drains. *British Journal of Hospital Medicine* **45**: 383–386.

Landis S, Murray T, Bolden S, Wingo PA (1998) Cancer statistics. *CA: A Cancer Journal for Clinicians* **48**: 6.

Light RW (1995) *Pneumothorax in pleural diseases*, 3rd edn. Williams and Wilkins, Baltimore.

Luketich JD *et al.* (1998) Chest tube insertion: a prospective evaluation of pain management. *Clinical Journal of Pain* **14**: 152–154.

Maddaus M, Ginsberg RJ (1995) Cancer/diagnosis and staging. In: Pearson FG, Deslauriers J, Ginsberg RJ *et al.* (eds) *Thoracic surgery*. Churchill Livingstone, New York.

Melton LJ, Hepper NCG, Offord KP (1979) Incidence of spontaneous pneumothorax in Olmstead County, Minnesota 1950–1974. *American Review of Respiratory Disease* **29**: 1379–1382.

Mountain CF (1997) Revisions in the international system for staging lung cancer. *Chest* **111**: 1710.

Mulshine ML, Tockman MS (1992) Considerations in population based screening for the early detection of lung cancer. In: Bernal SD, Hesketh PJ (eds) *Lung cancer differentiation: implications for diagnosis and treatment*. Marcel Decker, New York.

Selby C (2002) *Respiratory medicine: an illustrated colour text*. Churchill Livingstone, Edinburgh.

Sheppard FA, Ginsberg RJ, Feld R *et al.* (1991) Surgical treatment of limited small cell lung cancer. University of Toronto Oncology Group Experience. *Journal of Thoracic and Cardiovascular Surgery* **101**: 385–393.

Shields TW (1994) Lung cancer: etiology, carcinogenesis, molecular biology and pathology. In: Shields TW (ed.) *General thoracic surgery*, 4th edn. Williams & Wilkins, Baltimore.

Sridhar KS, Raub WA (1992) Present and past smoking history and other predisposing factors in 100 lung cancer patients. *Chest* **101**: 19.

Treasure T, Murphy JP (1989) *Pneumothorax Surgery* **75**: 1780–1786.

Wait MA, Sharma S, Hohn J *et al.* (1997) A randomized controlled trial of empyema therapy. *Chest* **111**: 1548–1551.

Respiratory Infection

7

Respiratory illness is the most common reason why the population consult their General Practitioners (BTS 2002). Almost a third (31%) of the population of England and Wales consulted their GP for a respiratory condition at least once during the year (1991–1992); this was three times higher than for cardiovascular conditions and twice as high as for musculoskeletal conditions (RCGP survey cited in BTS 2002).

The Royal College of General Practitioners (RCGP) survey further identified that the prevalence of respiratory disease is highest in children with two-thirds of children aged under five visiting their GP with a respiratory condition each year.

In comparison with the RCGP survey of 1981–1982, there has been an increase in the prevalence of respiratory disorders of 14%. While there has been a significant increase in the recorded incidence of asthma and COPD, in part due to a general agreement to adopt standard diagnostic methods, this rise fails to account for the steepness noted in the overall increased rate of occurrence of respiratory disorders. Respiratory infections such as tuberculosis (TB) have also shown a dramatic increase; in 2000 there were 5025 cases of TB reported to the Public Health Laboratory service, and this was a rise of 22% above the annual reported cases of TB during the 1990s.

The aims of this chapter include:
❑ To review the aetiology and treatment of common respiratory tract infections including:
the common cold;
pharyngitis;
sinusitis;
bronchitis;

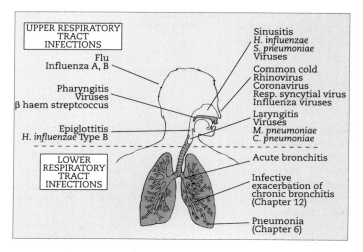

Fig. 7.1 Acute respiratory infections. With permission from Blackwell Publishing (Bourke 2003).

pneumonia;

tuberculosis.

❏ To consider the implications of the increased prevalence of TB and pneumonia within the UK.

❏ To review health care professional responsibilities and role in the management of these respiratory infections.

COMMON COLD

The common cold is one of the major causes of morbidity worldwide. In the United States it is responsible for the loss of 30 000 000 working days per year (Bartlett 2001) and results in over $1 billion per year spent on non-prescription remedies.

A number of conditions can cause symptoms of the common cold, but the name 'common cold' is usually reserved for those symptoms caused by an upper respiratory tract viral infection. The viruses that can cause colds include: *rhinovirus*; *corona-*

viruses; *adenovirus*; *parainfluenza* virus; RSV (respiratory syncy-tial virus) and *influenza* virus. Influenza causes common cold symptoms, but usually has a profound systemic response so that 'flu' is usually distinguishable from a 'cold'. RSV is an important cause of potentially serious disease in children, in the elderly and in immunocompromised patients.

Transmission of the viruses that cause the common cold is pri-marily by direct contact with respiratory secretions, usually by hand contact with an infected individual or contaminated object followed by self-inoculation by either finger to nose or finger to eye spread (Gwaltney and Hendley 1983). Aerosol spread appears important in the transmission of influenza virus (Bartlett 2001).

Symptoms of the common cold are well known to everyone. The incubation period is usually 2–4 days; initial symptoms include rhinorrhea, sneezing, nasal obstruction and postnasal drip. Other common symptoms include sore throat, throat clear-ing, hoarseness and cough, general malaise and low-grade fever.

Few conditions in medicine have so many therapeutic options that do not work. Those with probable benefit are largely limited to the administration of intranasal ipratropium bromide and analgesics. Intranasal ipratropium bromide has been demonstrated in clinical trials to reduce nasal drainage; it pro-duces a better outcome when initiated within 1 day following onset of symptoms (Hayden *et al.* 1996). Analgesics may help with the malaise and low-grade pyrexia and decongestants may help with sleeping, since nasal blocking can cause sleep disturbances.

Complications can occur with the common cold. One type of response consists of infections at contiguous sites that are often caused by bacteria, such as sinusitis, otitis media, bronchitis and pneumonia. The second form of response is related to chronic lung diseases; common colds are associated with exacerbations of chronic obstructive pulmonary disease, asthma and obstruc-tive sleep apnoea.

Preventing or decreasing the spread of the common cold is by avoidance of contact, especially hand contact with people exhibiting typical symptoms. Extra vitamin C was advocated as a method to prevent colds, but in clinical trials has not been proven to be of any benefit (Miller *et al.* 1977).

PHARYNGITIS

Pharyngitis may occur in isolation or as part of the common cold syndrome. Most pharyngitis is as a result of viral infection, but it may also be caused by agents, for example, group *A β-haemolytic streptococci* or *Mycoplasma pneumoniae*.

The patient complains of a sore throat, and there is erythema of the pharynx often with enlargement of the tonsils. Antibiotic therapy is rarely required since the disease is usually self-limiting (Bourke 2003). However the complications of severe streptococcal pharyngitis include otitis, sinusitis, peritonsillar abscesses and in rare cases osteomyelitis. In the developed world these are relatively rare due to rapid diagnosis and treatment following identification of causal organism (Bartlett 2001).

Methods adopted to limit the spread of infection centre around stratagems to promote the avoidance/isolation of those individuals with pharyngitis. There is a low risk associated upon exposure to those who are asymptomatic carriers.

SINUSITIS

Infection of the maxillary sinuses causes facial pain, nasal obstruction and discharge. Acute bacterial sinusitis is usually a complication secondary to the common cold. Symptoms can then overlap, and thus distinguishing between viral and bacterial sinusitis is usually based upon the existence of symptoms for more than one week. Often the patient experiences pain on one side of the face more severely than the other and will state that they felt better a few days after the onset of symptoms, but then become unwell again. This sequence of symptoms is due firstly to the onset of a cold, which is then followed by the secondary infection of bacterial sinusitis.

The goals of treatment are to: eradicate bacteria from the sinuses; prevent chronic sinusitis; prevent central nervous system, orbital and respiratory complications; and to relieve symptoms. The usual therapy includes empirically selected antibiotics combined with nasal decongestants.

CROUP

Croup is usually caused by a viral infection, such as RSV, parainfluenza virus, and rhinovirus. It is usually a childhood disease characterised by a harsh barking cough, which may progress to stridor. Often no treatment is necessary but some children develop severe lower respiratory infections and progressive respiratory distress requiring intubation and ventilation. Oral prednisolone is sometimes helpful in severe croup as is nebulised high-dose budesonide.

ACUTE EPIGLOTTITIS

Epiglottitis is a serious life-threatening disease usually caused by virulent strains of *Haemophilus influenzae* type B. Death results from occlusion of the airway by the inflamed epiglottis. Most common in children aged 2–3 years, but does occur in adults. Symptoms include pyrexia, sore throat, laryngitis and painful dysphagia. Symptoms of upper airway obstruction may develop rapidly with stridor and respiratory distress.

Treatment is usually the admission to hospital, commencement of antibiotic therapy and the examination of the upper airway (**only to be carried out where equipment for intubation and ventilation exist**).

INFLUENZA

Acute illness characterised by pyrexia, malaise, myalgia, headache and prostration together with upper respiratory symptoms. It is highly infectious and usually self-limiting, but can cause considerable morbidity and secondary illnesses such as sinusitis, otitis media and bacterial pneumonia. Older people, young children and those with underlying cardiac or respiratory disease are at greatest risk of death resulting from contraction of the influenza virus.

Treatment is usually based upon symptoms presented, with analgesia for myalgia and pyrexia and antibiotic therapy given in cases of secondary bacterial infection.

Influenza vaccine

This vaccine is prepared each year using the various strains of influenza believed likely to be prevalent in that year. The vaccine contains inactivated virus and gives between 70 and 80% effective protection against infection. When infection does occur it is usually less severe and associated with less morbidity than that found in unvaccinated patients.

Vaccination is carried out annually and is recommended for those with chronic respiratory conditions, chronic heart disease, renal failure, diabetes mellitus, and immunosuppression and for elderly people living in nursing homes.

ACUTE BRONCHITIS

This is infection of the trachea and bronchi, often caused by viruses. Symptoms include cough, mucus production, pyrexia and malaise. Acute bronchitis usually resolves spontaneously. Occasionally opportunistic bacterial secondary infections will occur which require treatment by a broad-spectrum antibiotic.

CHRONIC BRONCHITIS

Viruses are again the most common cause of exacerbations of chronic bronchitis. However bacterial infections are quite common with *Haemophilus influenzae* being the most commonly encountered (BTS 1997).

Symptoms include increased wheeze, increased dyspnoea, increased sputum volumes, and increased sputum purulence, chest tightness and fluid retention, and worsening of previous stable condition. Treatment is usually by broad-spectrum antibiotics: amoxicillin, oxytetracycline, ampicillin and cephalosporins may be considered. Patient assessment needs to be carried out to review whether it is possible to treat the patient in their home or if they require hospital admission. NICE (2004) have provided a simple chart to aid in the assessment of whether the patient should be treated at home or in a hospital environment.

Prevention

Those with chronic bronchitis should be advised not to smoke, have the influenza annual vaccination, and avoid exposure to inhospitable weather, which may exacerbate their symptoms.

PNEUMONIA

This is a significant cause of morbidity and mortality world-wide, with approximately 5 million children under the age of five dying worldwide as a consequence of pneumonia (Farr 1997). In the UK 1 in 1000 of the population are admitted to hospital each year with pneumonia, the disease causing 3000 deaths per year in the age group 15–55 years. In the older population 25% of all deaths are related to pneumonia (Bourke 2003; Obaro *et al.* 1996). Based upon 1992–1993 prices, community-acquired pneumonia incurred a direct healthcare cost of £441 million annually (BTS 2001). Consequently extensive and exhaustive guidelines on the treatment of community-acquired pneumonia have been produced worldwide; of specific note in the UK are the relevant guidelines published by the British Thoracic Society (2001).

Pneumonia is a general term indicating inflammation of the gas exchange region of the lungs; usually it implies parenchymal lung inflammation caused by infection. Pneumonia is either acquired in the community, either in a previously fit and well individual or in those who have a concomitant disease such as COPD or asthma. Hospital-acquired pneumonia is defined as a pneumonia developing two or more days after admission to hospital for another cause.

Symptoms include: cough, purulent sputum, fever, pleuritic chest pain and dyspnoea. There may be a history of upper respiratory tract infection, however this is not always the case. The initial phase of pneumonia may not have a productive cough associated with it. Atypical pneumonias may also lack the symptoms associated with a productive cough.

Investigations

Clinical investigations may aid in the diagnosis and provide some indication of the severity of the pneumonia. This is notoriously difficult and relies upon the experience of the practitioner and a full patient assessment. Localised chest sounds upon auscultation such as crackling or dullness may indicate pneumonia rather than bronchitis. Symptoms of severe respiratory distress (see Chapter 8) may be present and indicate the presence of a severe respiratory infection.

Initial clinical assessment thus focuses upon assessment of the patient and assessment of the severity of the disease. This provides clinical information that will aid in the location and commencement of treatment. Microbial investigations are indicated in all patients with pneumonia. This will identify a causal agent, aid in the delivering of appropriate treatment and eliminate other causes of this lung disease. Such investigations include sputum microscopy, culture and sensitivity, blood cultures, white cell count, pleural fluid microscopy culture and sensitivity, pneumococcal antigen tests and serological tests (Bourke 2003).

Treatment

Mild pneumonia in a fit patient can usually be treated at home, with broad-spectrum antibiotic therapy, mild analgesia and encouragement to maintain a healthy diet and mobilise frequently. Admission to hospital should be considered for those who do not have support at home or other social circumstances that indicate they cannot cope at home.

For severity assessment used to determine the management of community-acquired pneumonia in the community, see Fig. 7.2.

Severe pneumonia indicates admission to hospital. Appropriate treatment should be commenced to relieve the symptoms of respiratory distress; thus oxygen therapy should be used so that PaO_2 should be kept above 8 kPa and peripheral oxygen saturation above 90%. Intravenous fluid therapy should be initiated, diet should be reviewed and chest physiotherapy should be considered. Antibiotic therapy should be commenced and observation of the patient should be continuous to check for any alteration in the patient's condition. Admission to ITU is not uncommon in acute pneumonias since respiratory failure can occur rapidly in severe cases (Baudouin 2002).

After the commencement of antibiotic therapy, often used together with any adjuncts to aid the functioning of the respiratory system, improvement in the patient's condition usually occurs within several days.

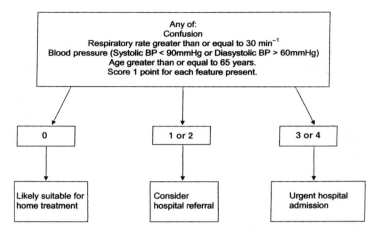

Fig. 7.2 Severity assessment used to determine management of pneumonia. With permission from Blackwell Publishing (Bourke 2003).

Prevention and risk

Prevention of pneumonia is non-specific but includes reducing poverty, poor nutrition, poor housing, smoking tobacco, and alcohol consumption (Woodhead *et al.* 1987). Underlying cardiorespiratory disease also increases the predisposition to pneumonia, as does age (the very young or the very old).

Pneumococcal vaccination is recommended by the Department of Health for all those aged 2 years or older in whom pneumococcal infection is likely to be more common or serious. However there is no evidence that the vaccination is likely to prevent community-acquired pneumonia in those patients designated in 'at risk groups' (NICE 2004).

TUBERCULOSIS (TB)

This is a common notifiable infectious disease; the World Health Organization (WHO) in 1993 declared TB a global emergency. WHO estimates that 1.72 billion people have latent infection with mycobacterium tuberculosis, 15–20 million people have active disease and 3 million deaths occur each year from TB (Bourke 2003; Sudre *et al.* 1992).

Notification rates in England and Wales reached a low of circa 5000 a year in 1987, but are once again increasing (BTS 2000b). This is mainly seen in inner-city areas, with a high risk of TB found among the homeless, drug misusers, alcoholics, those with HIV, and ethnic minorities. The clinical course of TB often evolves over many years, and represents a complex interaction between the infecting organism (*Mycobacterium tuberculosis*) and the infected person. TB has two infectious phases: firstly the primary infection with tubercule bacilli and then the development of active smear-positive TB.

Primary infection

Infection occurs as a result of inhalation of the organisms from an infected individual. Soon after the primary infection enters the lung, the inflammatory response occurs and a calcified lesion is left. This is visible upon chest X-ray. This stage of the disease may be asymptomatic, or there may be mild symptoms including mild febrile illness, erythema nodosum (painful indurated shin lesions) and small pleural effusions. However the disease may progress in this stage causing lung consolidation and bronchiectasis (Ward *et al.* 2002). Blood-borne spread of this disease may cause miliary tuberculosis (widespread infection involving many tissues) and the lethal complication of tuberculosis meningitis. Infection spread in this initial stage may lie dormant in any organ of the body for many years only to reactivate later.

Post-primary tuberculosis

This is the pattern of the disease seen after the development of specific immunity. It may occur as a consequence of re-exposure to the infection (inhalation once again of *Mycobacterium tuberculosis*), re-activation of the disease or direct progression of the illness from the primary stage.

It usually occurs over months and symptoms include malaise, anorexia, weight loss, night sweats and productive cough. Clinical signs of pneumonia and pleural effusion are common.

Reactivation occurs as a result of decreased immunity within the host; consequently it often occurs in old age, in the immune compromised individuals and in those with other co-morbidities. The lungs are the most usual site of post-primary disease, especially the apexes. Table 7.1 illustrates some of the common sites and consequences of infection from TB.

Table 7.1 Common sites and treatment options for TB (Omerod 1998).

Symptoms	Major organs affected	Treatment options
Respiratory symptoms. Upper lobe pneumonia, malaise, weight loss and cough are prominent	Lungs	6-month regimen comprising rifampicin, isoniazid, pyrazinamide and ethambutol for initial two months followed by rifampicin and isoniazid for further four months (BTS 1998).
Painless lymph node enlargement	Peripheral lymph nodes	6-month drug regimen as recommended for respiratory TB disease.
Bone destruction occurs without new bone formation, deformation, pain and potential nerve entrapment	Bone and joints	Ambulatory chemotherapy usually effective, occasionally surgery may be required. 6-month treatment used in treatment of respiratory TB.
Chest pain, shortness of breath, reduced exercise tolerance	Pericarditis	6-month treatment as for respiratory TB.
Comparable to meningococcal meningitis. Coma, fits, hydrocephalus	TB meningitis	Chemotherapy should be chosen which penetrates cerebrospinal fluid well.
Miliary TB low-grade fever, steady patient decline	Symptoms will depend upon tissue and organ involvement	Respiratory TB treatment usually adequate unless CNS involvement in which case chemotherapy should be carefully chosen.

One of the major problems with the treatment of TB is the duration that the chemotherapy occurs. This can lead to issues with poor patient compliance and the re-occurrence of TB resistant to the standard therapy. In order to reduce this it is essential that the patients are fully aware of the consequences of TB infection, the public health risk and the aims of chemotherapy treatment.

Directly observed therapy (DOT) is recommended for those patients that may find compliance with therapeutic regimen difficult (Morse 1996). This involves observation of the ingestion of every dose of medication by an external witness. Conflict can occur in this case between the civil rights of the individual and the public health issues; however the aim is to engender co-operation and not to seek dissent and poor compliance.

Control and prevention of TB

All confirmed and suspected cases of TB must be notified to an appropriate appointed officer. It is well documented that under notification occurs (Ferguson *et al.* 1998; Sheldon *et al.* 1992). Notification will trigger contact tracing which is essential to ascertain and identify those at risk of developing the disease and offer preventative measures such as BCG, or to identify those with early asymptomatic disease and commence appropriate therapy. It will also provide surveillance data and thus aid in the planning and support of appropriate health care services.

Organisation of local TB services should be based upon a local written policy (BTS 2000a), outlining all the TB prevention and control measures that are in place in the local area. All patients with TB should be under the care of health professionals who are adequately trained in the treatment and management of TB (BTS 1998).

Treatment of TB should be undertaken in the patient's home whenever possible (BTS 2000b); however some patients will require hospital admission. Patients with non-pulmonary TB can be nursed on open wards; those with pulmonary TB should be nursed in single rooms with air vented to the outside. Some environments can provide 'negative pressure' rooms until risk assessments can be made based upon sputum samples and the active status of the TB. Visiting, including the visits involving young children, should be limited to those who have already been exposed to the risk of TB (BTS 2000). The risk to staff is low if they attend the patient in a routine manner. Any staff who have been exposed to patients with undiagnosed respiratory TB should be treated as close contacts of the patient and subsequently followed up. Detailed advice can be found in the report 'Control and prevention of tuberculosis in the United Kingdom, 2000' (BTS).

Contact tracing

Contact tracing is undertaken for the following reasons:

- To detect associated cases.
- To detect persons infected without disease symptoms.
- To identify candidates for BCG vaccination.
- To detect source case.
- To screen local population with high incidence of TB and prompt further investigation.

Contact tracing requires the resources of many health care professionals and should be carried out under the overarching local policy agreed for TB management.

Prevention of TB

The provision of good nutrition, adequate sanitation, less crowded housing, fresh air, tuberculin testing of herds and pasteurisation of milk were all identified and utilised as effective measures in the prevention and treatment of TB prior to the availability of effective chemotherapy for the cure. They are still recognised as minimal cost stratagems that are fundamental, effective and essential in the prevention and control of TB in large urban populations.

Vaccination

The injection of attenuated Bacille Calmette-Guérin (BCG) intradermally provokes a T-cell mediated immune response, which activates the destruction of macrophages laden with mycobacteria upon any subsequent intracellular infection. It is variably effective, with less effect noticed against the eastern Africa forms of TB (Selby 2002). Widespread vaccination in the UK has helped in the reduction of TB, and it remains the policy to offer BCG vaccination to all children aged 13–14 years in the UK, although this is under review (BTS 2000b).

Skin testing

Intradermal injection of a purified protein derivative (PPD) of *Mycobacterium tuberculin* is administered either as a single multiple injection Heaf test, or a Mantoux test by a series of single injections with increasing doses of PPD. The skin reaction 3–7 days later is measured as either the pattern of skin response to the multi-injected test or the extent of skin indication to sequential Mantoux injections.

A test is used prior to BCG vaccination to identify those who would not benefit; it may also identify those with an excessive response suggestive of a recent infection. However it has limited value in the diagnosis of TB since time delay, previous BCG vaccination, or intercurrent illness will also influence the result.

Health professionals have a responsibility to reduce the burden of respiratory infection upon the health service and the

Table 7.2 Reading a Heaf test.

Grade	Description	Indication
0	From nothing to feeling no more than 3 raised red spots.	Negative; no previous immunological experience.
1	4–6 separate raised red spots.	Weak reaction, previous 0 environmental mycobacteria infection or weak response to BCG.
2	6 raised spots forming a circle.	Previous infection of BCG response.
3	Coalescence with raised centre.	Previous event recent, infection may have been subclinical.
4	Blisters	Previous even recent infection may have been subclinical.

welfare state. By increasing vigilance and early diagnosis it is possible to reduce the impact of some of these illnesses upon the patient and their families.

Prevention is always better than cure and this should be the main focus of health education provided. The importance of this is exemplified in contact tracing those who may have been exposed to TB and virulent pneumonia.

SUMMARY

❏ Respiratory infections are a major cause of health service utilisation.

❏ Pneumonia is often under-diagnosed and is a major cause of mortality, especially in those patients who are over 65 years of age or who have other co-morbidities.

❏ TB has once again become an increasing problem in the UK; it has a significant morbidity and mortality associated with it.

❏ Worldwide, TB affects one-third of the population (Selby 2002).

❏ Health professionals have a duty to treat the symptoms of respiratory infections in the correct manner. This depends upon the accurate and appropriate assessment of the patient and then the implementation of suitable care.

REFERENCES

Baudouin SV (2002) Critical care management of community acquired pneumonia. *Thorax* **57**: 267–271.

Bartlett JG (2001) *Management of respiratory tract infections*, 3rd edn. Lippincott Williams & Wilkins, Philadelphia.

Bourke SJ (2003) *Respiratory medicine*, 6th edn. Blackwell Publishing, Oxford.

BTS (1998) Chemotherapy and management of tuberculosis in the United Kingdom: recommendations. *Thorax* **53**: 536–548.

BTS COPD Guidelines Group of Standards of Care Committee of the BTS (1997) BTS Guidelines for the Management of COPD. *Thorax* **52** (Suppl. 5): S1–S28.

BTS (2000a) Management of opportunistic mycobacterial infections: Joint Tuberculosis Committee Guidelines 1999. *Thorax* **55**: 210–218.

BTS (2000b) Control and prevention of tuberculosis in the United Kingdom: Code of Practice 2000. *Thorax* **55**: 887–901.

BTS (2001) BTS guidelines for the management of community acquired pneumonia in adults. *Thorax* **56**: Suppl. iv1–64.

BTS (2002) The burden of lung disease. *Epidemiology* **107**: 357.

Farr B (1997) Prognosis and decisions in pneumonia. *New England Journal of Medicine* **336** (4): 228–289.

Ferguson A, Bennett D, Conning S (1998) Notification of tuberculosis in patients with AIDS. *Journal of Public Health Medicine* **20**: 218–220.

Gwaltney JM, Hendley JO (1983) Rhinovirus colds: epidemiology, clinical characteristics and transmission. *European Journal of Respiratory Disease* **64** (Suppl. 128): 336.

Hayden FG, Diamond L, Wood PB *et al.* (1996) Effectiveness and safety of intranasal ipratropium bromide in common colds. *Annals of Internal Medicine* **125**: 89.

Miller JZ, Nance WE, Norton JA *et al.* (1977) Therapeutic effect of vitamin C: a co-twin control study. *JAMA* **237**: 248.

Morse DI (1996) Directly observed therapy for tuberculosis. *British Medical Journal* **312**: 719–720.

NICE (2004) COPD national guideline on management of chronic obstructive pulmonary disease in adults in primary and secondary care. *Thorax* **59** (Suppl. 1): 1–232.

Obaro SK, Monteil MA, Henderson DC (1996) The pneumococcal problem. *British Medical Journal* **312**: 1521–1525.

Ormerod LP (1998) Chemotherapy and management of tuberculosis in the United Kingdom: British Thoracic Society Guidelines. *Thorax* **53**: 536–548.

Selby C (2002) *Respiratory medicine*. Churchill Livingstone, Edinburgh.

Sheldon CD, King K, Cock H *et al.* (1992) Notification of tuberculosis: how many cases are never reported? *Thorax* **47**: 1015–1018.

Sudre P, Dam G, Kochi A (1992) Tuberculosis: a global overview of the situation today. *Bulletin of the WHO* **70**: 149–159.

Taylor D (1996) Tuberculosis: knowledge and practice. *Nursing Times* **92** (42): 1–4.

Ward JPT, Ward J, Wiener CM, Leach RM (2003) *The respiratory system at a glance*. Blackwell Publishing, Oxford.

Woodhead MA, MacFarlane JT, McCracken JS, Rose DH, Finch RG (1987) Prospective study of the aetiology and outcome of pneumonia in the community. *Lancet* **I**: 671–674.

www.brit-thoracic.org/Guidelines for the management of community acquired pneumonia updated 30.04.04.

Respiratory Assessment   **8**

Correct and structured assessments of patients are the crucial underpinning necessary for the efficient planning of clinical care (Woodrow 2002). This is true for all clinical situations; however in situations of respiratory distress rapid assessment and monitoring are also essential (Kendrick *et al.* 2000). The speed of that initial response can be considered to be the critical factor in the delivery of the prompt intervention necessary to save life.

This chapter aims to:
- ❏ Outline principles of respiratory assessment.
- ❏ Review the principles of blood gas analysis.
- ❏ Explain principles and use of pulse oximetry.
- ❏ Explain the basic use of spirometry and peak flow meters.
- ❏ Consider the common respiratory health status assessment questionnaires.
- ❏ Consider the importance of correct and appropriate documentation.

PRINCIPLES OF RESPIRATORY ASSESSMENT

Chapter 5 considered the assessment of patients with respect to the commencement and cessation of oxygen therapy. This chapter will discuss how to carry out a more detailed assessment and evaluation of the patient's respiratory function, and consider some of the effects of aging upon respiratory physiology.

Useful information can be gained about the respiratory function simply by observing a patient objectively. It is important to note that if clinical observation reveals respiratory distress, then the duties and responsibilities of a qualified nurse are to ensure that this problem is addressed immediately, even at the cost of discontinuing the planned respiratory assessment (The NMC Code of Conduct, 2000). It is a reasonable and natural assumption to expect both registered and non-registered health professionals to notify qualified practitioners as soon as they observe any patient in respiratory distress. There are clinically clear, recognisable symptoms of severe respiratory distress. For example, a patient who is found to be unable to complete sentences is displaying such a symptom (BTS 2003) and this must evoke a prompt response. There are however situations, most commonly found with the youngest patients, where it may be difficult to know whether a new patient has problems in completing sentences under normal circumstances. With such cases the inability or reluctance of the patient to eat or drink should be regarded as possibly due to dyspnoea, and it should be regarded clinically as a possible sign of severe respiratory distress.

OBSERVATION OF A PATIENT
This will yield information concerning:

- Respiration rate.
- Respiration depth.
- Respiration pattern (rhythm), use of accessory muscles of respiration.
- Skin colour.
- Physical condition, unkempt appearance, possible malnourishment.
- Presence of coughing, whether productive or not.
- Sounds of breathing.

Respiration rate
For fit, healthy adults with no respiratory or cardiac disease *the respiration rate at rest* is usually 10–14 breaths per minute (Darovic 1997); however Torrance and Elley (1996) suggest that the *respiration rate at rest for adults* should be less than 12 breaths per minute. The presence of cardiac disease, respiratory illness and other illnesses especially those with an associated pyrexia

will often increase respiration rate. A rise in respiration rate is a sensitive indicator of a patient's deterioration (Goldhill White and Sumner 1999). It is thus an important clinical observation that indicates an altered homeostasis, which may or may not require clinical intervention. The gaseous exchange occurring in the alveoli of the elderly will have often become impaired, especially if there is a history of exposure to the effects of tobacco smoke. In this older population an increase in the resting respiration rate will not be uncommon. If no positive information is available on the normal respiration rate of an older debilitated patient, it becomes important to arrive at a best estimate before further clinical evaluation of the patient continues. All the moderating factors influencing respiration rate should enter into such estimations.

Tachypnoea (fast respiration rate) is usually indicative of the 'need' of the body to redress an oxygen deficit and/or reduce the carbon dioxide level in the blood. Tachypnoea will thus be observed in healthy athletes upon completion of short explosive athletic events, and be frequently met by the health-care professional when treating patients with: untreated COPD; end-stage COPD; acute severe asthma; lung cancer; cardiac disease and other respiratory crises. Tachypnoea if prolonged can lead to respiratory exhaustion and in some cases respiratory arrest. It is thus an observation that usually in a clinical situation triggers investigation and possible intervention.

Bradypnoea (low respiration rate) is usually caused by depression of the respiratory centres within the brain; this can be caused by the use of opiate medication or from clinical catastrophic events, such as a stroke. Bradypnoea can occur after a period of tachypnoea and this sequence of symptoms is often the forewarning of possible imminent respiratory arrest.

Respiration pattern

Normal subconscious control of breathing will maintain a reasonably regular rate and pattern of breathing. An irregular pattern (see Chapter 5) can result from brain damage, medication and especially by a conscious alteration of breathing patterns by the patient. Thus the annotation of respiratory pattern can sometimes provide preliminary information concerning the neurological status.

It is important to observe patients regularly and note any abnormal respiratory rate. Such regular observation does not always have to be carried out formally, in fact if patients are aware that their respiration is being observed they often alter their respiration pattern. Respiration rates can be observed and noted when carrying out other tasks such as taking blood pressures, pulse rate, making the bed, etc.

Respiration depth
Respiration depth is assessed indirectly by clinical observation. It can be a reasonable estimate of how much air is breathed in during each inspiration. At an appropriate point in the treatment of the patient information concerning tidal volume can be obtained directly using spirometry.

In fit healthy individuals the main respiratory muscles used in breathing are the diaphragm and intercostal muscles. Intercostal movement is easily visible whereas normal diaphragmatic movement is not easily observed. Laboured breathing, or dyspnoea will utilise accessory muscles to breathe; these include the abdominal muscles, the sternocleidomastoid and pectoral muscles. In older people the obvious use of the diaphragm and abdominal muscles to aid breathing is considered acceptable (Bennet 2002).

While the body is at rest, the respiratory muscles normally use only 1–3% of the total body oxygen available. In contrast the consequences of respiratory disease can increase that figure dramatically. The debility may result in the respiratory effort required to breath demanding a large expenditure of energy, with the metabolic pathways supplying that energy being judged to consume 25–30% of the total oxygen being made available to the body (Hinds & Watson 1996).

Skin colour
Skin colour can provide basic information concerning the efficiency and basic functioning of the respiratory system. The condition known as cyanosis is recognised by a bluish skin

colouring and is usually associated with hypoxia. It is seen most obviously in: nail-beds; the mucous membranes (e.g. lips and mouth); the tip of the nose and the earlobes (Darovic 1997). Cyanosis is in itself a good indicator that there is insufficient oxygen to maintain the saturation level of oxyhaemoglobin (oxygen bound to haemoglobin) at above 80%. Indirect or direct methods may be used to quantify the saturation level of oxyhaemoglobin in either arterial or capillary blood. However any observation of cyanosis indicates the presence of severe respiratory distress, which might have been prevented by earlier intervention.

Coughing

Coughing is a reflex action directed towards the removal of foreign bodies, for example bacteria trapped in mucus. Thus a persistent cough may indicate a chronic respiratory infection. Such coughs should be recorded in the notes with some annotation (strong/weak, dry, frequency, hoarse or barking, etc). Coughing can become very distressing so its relief is important.

Sputum production is a clinical feature of respiratory disease and the sputum should be observed for colour, consistency and quantity. Table 8.1 illustrates how the physical properties of sputum relate to several respiratory conditions.

With the use of a stethoscope, **normal breath sounds** should be bilateral and audible in all lung zones. **Noisy respiration** is clearly audible to the naked ear and is usually a sign of respi-

Table 8.1 Type of sputum (Jevon & Ewens 2001).

Consistency	Colour	Respiratory condition
Thick	Viscid	Severe asthma
Thin	Watery	Cardiac disease/emphysema
Mucoid	White	Asthma and chronic bronchitis
Purulent	Green, yellow	Infection
N/A	Blood	Carcinoma of the lung, or pulmonary embolism

ratory distress. **Stridor** is a high pitch sound usually occurring on inspiration. A **wheeze** is characterised by a noisy musical sound produced by the turbulent flow of air through the bronchi and bronchioles. Wheeze is often more pronounced on expiration and can be associated with asthma, chronic bronchitis and emphysema. A rattle in the chest indicates the presence of fluid (pulmonary oedema or sputum) in the upper airway. These sounds are all audible to the naked ear (Ahern & Philpot 2002, Jevon & Ewens 2001, Bennett 2002).

Physical condition

Does the patient appear exhausted, confused anxious or unresponsive? Are there any non-verbal expressions of pain observable, especially upon inspiration and expiration? What posture does the patient adopt? An erect posture often improves the symptoms of breathlessness, as do other commonly adopted positions include sitting up and resting forward arms extended over several pillows placed upon a table.

INFORMATION FROM THE PATIENT

This is an important component in the assessment of the patient, providing the quickest route to vital information on the past and present health status of the patient. During this assessment several issues need to be considered, namely, the severity of clinical condition at time of assessment and the possible need for immediate intervention. If the patient is in severe respiratory distress, then detailed information obtained from the patient will be limited. However there may be relatives or neighbours present or waiting outside the examination room, who may be able to give succinct objective answers and can certainly provide useful background information. When verbal methods are being used in the assessment of the acutely breathless patient it may be helpful to use closed questions initially to gain rapid information. However the continued and protracted use of closed questions in the assessment of patients is not generally advocated.

Experienced practitioners will have already established a systematic order to gain information from the patient, and will be adaptable in their approach. For example by utilising the information the patient volunteers gratuitously in general conversation often reveals much about the patient's quality of life and general lifestyle. This background may well help to focus further questions and elicit rapidly the conditions leading up to the present respiratory crisis. However the younger relatively less experienced practitioners may find the following order initially helpful in obtaining and recording the necessary data (Barkauskas *et al.* 1994).

1. Biographical information.
2. Patient's reason for seeking care (main complaint).
3. Present health and present illness status.
4. Past health history/problems.
5. Current health history.
6. Family health history.
7. Review of systems: physical systems; functional systems; sociological system; psychological system.
8. Developmental data.
9. Nutritional data.

To expand on these further:

- **Demographic information.** Include name, age, gender, address, telephone number; race; religion; marital status; occupation (present and past); contact details of next of kin; source of referral (Emergency, GP, etc.). Ensure that this information is written legibly, dated and the source of information clearly stated, i.e. from patient or other source. Include your own contact information in case of any queries later.
- **Present health/illness status.** Describes why the patient seeks care. Includes details of usual health; symptoms in chronological order including onset (date); manner gradual or sudden; duration; precipitating factors, frequency of symptoms since onset; patterns of remission; alleviating and/or aggravating factors; relevant family information.
- **Past health history.** Include past general health, childhood illnesses, accidents, hospitalisations; past surgery; acute and chronic illnesses; allergies.

- **Current health information.** Include the current medication and assess compliance with regimen; use of tobacco; alcohol; caffeine; illegal drugs; self-prescribed medications; exercise patterns; sleep patterns. Allergies should be identified and causal agent noted, together with any allergic response and therapies that relieve the reaction.
- **Family health history.** It is accepted that nature and nurture are both important components in determining the susceptibility to many diseases and illnesses. This is frequently referred to as a family 'trait'. Many respiratory conditions have a genetic component to them, e.g. asthma, cystic fibrosis. Other illnesses appear to potentiate respiratory illness, e.g. cardiac disease. In any assessment and prognosis such 'traits' and known triggers should not be understated nor underestimated. Respiratory illness may be life-limiting (e.g. COPD) and patients may need the physical, financial and emotional support of their family. It is clearly of direct importance to long-term care of the patient, to make some assessment of the health status of other family members and provide additional health care support when and where necessary.
- **Review of systems.** This may be left to a medical colleague; however the principle is as follows: assess the functioning of each physiological system from head to toe. Checklists are often invaluable.
- **Nutritional assessment.** This should include the average daily food intake and the documentation of the body mass index (see Chapter 3).

PHYSIOLOGICAL ASSESSMENT

Palpation and percussion of the thorax are sophisticated skills used in respiratory assessment. They involve the use of hands and fingers to gather information through the senses of touch and hearing. More information can be obtained from Cox (1997); Seidal *et al.* (1995) and Ruch (1999).

Chest auscultation is also a sophisticated skill; however it is commonly used by many health professionals and should be considered in more detail. Auscultation (listening via the aid of usually a stethoscope) to the chest can provide accurate and diagnostic information on the condition of the heart, lungs and pleura. Patients should be fully informed about the procedure and their consent and privacy ensured. The patient should be in a sitting position if possible allowing access to the anterior, posterior and lateral regions of the thorax. To facilitate an improvement in the ability to clearly distinguish the breath sounds, it is important to try and reduce all sources of extraneous sounds, such as rustling bed covers, talking relatives, etc. Figure 8.1 illustrates the sequence for listening to the thorax; this should be undertaken by placing either the diaphragm or the bell of the stethoscope on the patient's skin and listening to both inspiration and expiration. Comparison should be made between right and left sides of the thorax, with the stethoscope placed at similar locations.

Normal breath sounds are described in Table 8.2, but there are many other breath sounds that can be heard and as clinical experience increases it becomes easier to differentiate between normal and abnormal. The primary aim of this chapter is to

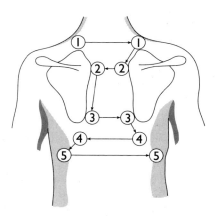

Fig. 8.1 Chest auscultation. With permission from Blackwell Publishing (Cox 2004).

197

Table 8.2 Normal breath sounds (Cox 1997).

Sound	Intensity of expiration	Pitch of expiration	Duration of inspiration and expiration	Location
Bronchial	Usually high	High	Expiration longer than inspiration	Trachea
Broncho-vesicular	Medium	Medium	Inspiration and expiration equal	Near the bronchi below the clavicles and between the scapulae, especially on the right side
Vesicular	Soft	Low	Inspiration longer than expiration	Healthy lung

introduce the normal breath sounds heard upon auscultation, thus any sounds that are not normal must warrant further investigation and consultation with other health professionals. To gain further experience ask for help and training from suitable health professionals.

Pulse oximetry

The basic technology has been available for over 50 years, although its general and widespread use in clinical practice did not occur until the early 1990s. The rapid advances in all areas of digital technology have led to the development of more robust systems that are easier to use, smaller in size, quicker, more accurate, with better displays and relatively cheaper. Their use and potential is now readily accepted by all the health professionals. However, despite their widespread use Stoneham *et al.* (1994) revealed a widespread lack of knowledge concerning accurate and appropriate use of pulse oximeters.

Pulse oximeters measure both pulse rate and the level of haemoglobin oxygen saturation in the peripheral arterial blood. They are reasonably accurate to within +/−3%. However their accuracy depends on good practice and they should be regularly re-calibrated as indicated by the manufacturer's protocol. Despite their improved robustness they should be protected from the risks associated with careless handling.

Pulse oximeters work by transmitting red and infrared light through body tissue, such as fingertips, earlobes, etc. Most of the light emitted by the probe is absorbed by the body tissue. The light that is transmitted through the tissue is detected by the photoelectric sensors found on the face of the other side of the probe. The microchip is programmed to calculate the haemoglobin saturation by the application of de Beer's Law.

Oxygen-rich haemoglobin and oxygen poor haemoglobin have different and quite specific absorption spectra giving rise to the well-known bright red colour of oxygen rich haemoglobin in arterial blood. The absorption of the oxygen rich and oxygen poor haemoglobin can be measured and the difference of absorption between full capillaries (systole) and empty ones (diastole), produces a difference in the that enables microchip calculation of haemoglobin saturation. This measurement is repeated over at least five pulses (Harrahill 1991). A caveat must be applied: since the pulse is only measured at the probe site it may not accurately reflect the heart rate, for example atrial fibrillation can cause inaccurate pulse oximetry.

The pulse oximetry reading should only be accepted for critical consideration if the following conditions apply: the wave form obtained on the screen should be as in Fig. 8.2. This demonstrates a clear trace with a well defined wave form. A bar graph will also display as a series of rectangles. These rectangles should fill the graph if the pulse is adequate (Fig. 8.3). The exact number and shape of the rectangles varies between manufacturers; however the underlying principle is the same for each oximeter.

The following limitations are clearly understood to apply to pulse oximetry. Saturation (S) is measured in peripheral (p) capillaries; hence it is the saturation of peripheral oxygen (SpO_2). In health this should *reflect* the arterial saturation of oxygen SaO_2; however SaO_2 per se is not measured by pulse oximetry, but upon arterial blood gas analysis.

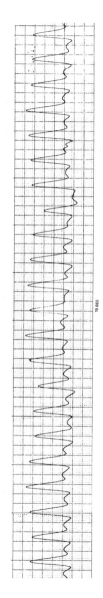

Fig. 8.2 Wave form from pulse oximetry. With permission from Blackwell Publishing (Jevon 2002).

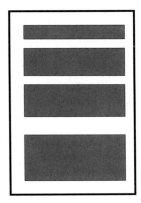

Fig. 8.3 Bar graph from pulse oximetry.

Respiratory failure is usually considered to exist in adults when pulse oximetry reveals SpO_2 less than 90% (Woodrow 1999); however in children this 'clinical alert' figure is usually set at the higher SpO_2 value of not less than 92%. Some patients in type II respiratory failure (see Chapter 5) will have become tolerant to a low SpO_2 for example 85–90%. These patients should be identified early and their 'atypical' pulse oximetry results documented clearly. This prevents undue anxiety and hasty intervention when a random SpO_2 results in a low reading.

Pulse oximeters have audible alarms and these alarms have a manufactured limit upon which they will respond; however it is better practice to set the alarm limits for each individual patient requiring continuous monitoring. Pulse oximeters also have an audible signal indicating the recognition of a pulse; in many cases this is turned off, but it can be useful in situations where the monitor screen cannot be seen, such as while carrying out other procedures (e.g. inserting a chest drain). However caution should be attached to any tendency to totally rely on this signal for assurance and it should never be the sole or principal method used to monitor the patient.

Factors that may alter pulse oximetry readings:

- Peripheral vasoconstriction.
- Dysrhythmias.
- Shivering (Stoneham *et al.* 1994).
- High bilirubin levels (Dobson 1993) will increase the absorption of the infrared and red light by body tissues.
- Dark skin.
- Dried blood.
- Black/blue nail varnish (Wahr & Temper 1996).
- Intravenous dyes (Fox 2002).
- External light (heat lamps, fluorescent lights (Ralston *et al.* 1992).
- Lower values of SpO_2 have a greater probability of being inaccurate.
- Carbon monoxide poisoning (Dobson 1993).

Peripheral pulse oximetry has the advantage of being painless for the patient while providing for the clinician a robust monitor that is accurate to within narrow limits; it has the merit of being relatively quick and easy to attach to accessible regions of the subject's body. It has a low infection risk and in clinics it can be used several times during the session since it can be cleaned between patients easily and effectively.

Arterial blood gas analysis can thus be reserved for those cases where more detailed results are required. Understanding the factors that influence the accuracy of the readings obtained from the pulse oximeter has become an essential part of the training of new health practitioners and will ensure that the patient receives the best care.

Pulse oximetry should be used as an aid in making clinical decisions; 'one off' readings are rarely useful and successive readings reveal more valuable information. However clinical observation and detailed patient assessment will help indicate if a patient who is normally fit and well has any overt or acute problem with an SpO_2 of 90%; as stated earlier this value is regarded as an acceptable SpO_2 in a patient diagnosed with type II respiratory failure.

ARTERIAL BLOOD GAS ANALYSIS

Arterial blood gas analysis provides accurate and reliable information pertaining to the patient's respiratory functioning, assuming that the sample is taken and then analysed appropriately.

Common sites for obtaining samples of arterial blood gas for analysis are: ear lobes; radial artery; femoral artery or via an arterial line inserted into the patient. Obtaining arterial blood directly from an artery is a painful procedure for the patient, necessitating the use of an arterial stab method. If this procedure for taking arterial blood is to be used, then good practice would recommend the use of local anaesthesia to reduce the pain (Hope *et al.* 1998). Arterial stabs are usually undertaken by the medically trained personnel; however the care of the patient before and after the procedure are the crucial roles that are the responsibility of the nurse. Once an artery has been pierced to obtain an arterial sample, the nurse usually has to place significant pressure upon the site to reduce the probability of an arterial bleed. This pressure should be maintained for a minimum of five minutes (Sheehy & Lombardi 1995); however clotting or bleeding disorders can significantly increase the length of time the nurse has to spend applying the necessary pressure.

Taking capillary blood from earlobes is less painful to the patient and the results are usually within 2% accuracy of an arterial stab (Pitkin *et al.* 1994).

Normal adult arterial blood gas results are illustrated in Table 8.3.

Table 8.3 Normal adult arterial blood gases.

Name	Normal values
PaO_2	12–14 kPa
$PaCO_2$	4.6–6.0 kPa
PH	7.35–7.45
HCO_3	22–26 mmol/L
SaO_2	95%+
Base excess	−2 to +2

Once arterial blood has been taken it should be analysed quickly. At normal room temperatures, gas exchange and metabolism will continue *in vitro* within the red blood cells and plasma. To minimise such degradation it is sometimes the practice to place the syringe with the arterial sample in a larger container of ice. Since this may cause damage to the syringe and thereby contaminate the blood sample, it is better to place the syringe in a container of iced water; this will then allow the arterial blood gas analysis to be reasonably accurate up to 60 minutes from the time the sample was taken (Clutton-Brock 1997). However requests for the analysis are always deemed to be urgent and the results become available soon after the sample has been taken.

Abnormal arterial blood gas results can be as a result of respiratory failure or other major physiological system failure such as renal failure. It is important to know the normal values and seek advice from more experienced practitioners if abnormal results are obtained.

Measurement of peak flow

Peak flow meters measure the peak flow (highest flow) of air on forced expiration and the value given is generally known as peak expiratory flow rate (PEFR). Clinically if larger airways are occluding, for example due to asthma, then patients cannot expire the air from their lungs with a high degree of force and velocity. A simple analogy to consider is to try blowing all the air out of your lungs through a straw. This would take a long time and is arduous. Repeat, but this time replace the straw with the cardboard tube of a kitchen roll. It is easier, faster and more comfortable to blow through the cardboard kitchen roll than a straw.

PEFR is dependent upon the age, gender and height of the individual. Standard reference values for PEFR have been generated (see Appendix A). However, they do not routinely consider ethnic differences that may be significant clinically.

Peak flow meters measure the rate of expiration of air from the lungs in litres per minute (L min^{-1}). 'Mini-Wright' and 'Wright' peak flow meters are used routinely in clinical practice.

These devices are for single patient use only and **must not** be used for multi-patients since they cannot be cleaned adequately enough to ensure there is no risk of transmitting prions (some prions are believed to be responsible for CJD). However, in some situations the use of disposable mouthpieces that contain one-way valves has been considered acceptable. These mouthpieces fit over the original mouthpiece of the meter. Their safety in general use is based upon the premise that these disposable mouthpieces are only used once and thus cannot transmit infections to the next patient. The manufacturers of the mouthpieces clearly state it is for single patient use only. All staff using disposable mouthpieces should be well-trained and totally compliant with the instructions. A note of caution must be given to this practice, since it only takes one person to forget to use a new disposable mouthpiece for this to fail. A system of double checking and immediately disposing of the mouthpiece after use should ensure complete safety.

Perhaps the only completely foolproof system however is to defer to the original meter manufacturer's recommendation that the apparatus is for single patient use only and ensure this is the observed practice.

September 1st 2004 saw the introduction of peak flow meters that have a logarithmic scale upon them, to conform to EU regulations. They are easily identified since the Mini-Wright peak flow meters have a yellow background to their scale.

How to use a peak flow meter
(See Fig. 8.4.)

Ideally always demonstrate this technique to the patient; however in some clinical areas this may not be possible.

1. Ask the patient to stand or sit up. If this is not possible try and get the patient into the most upright position possible.
2. Ask the patient to hold the peak flow meter horizontally and ensure that the gauge marker is at the bottom of the scale.
3. Get the patient to breathe in deeply, place their lips around the mouthpiece and form a tight seal.
4. Ask the patient to breathe out as quickly and hard as possible.

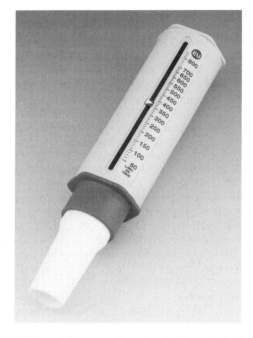

Fig. 8.4 Mini-Wright peak flow meter. Reproduced with permission from Clement Clark.

5. Read the position that the marker arrow has now reached and record this result.
6. Repeat steps 1–5 twice more.

The rational for repeating the test is that the patient is engaged in a certain amount of 'learning the technique', thus as they get better at it the result will improve. Their confidence will improve and thus they will expire more forcefully and fully. Any error in technique will be observed and corrected by the nurse.

Single peak flow readings are of limited use clinically (Kendrick & Smith 1992); however they can confirm the extent of respiratory distress. In asthma for example, if a patient is unable to achieve a peak flow reading of one-third of their best then according to the 2003 asthma treatment guidelines (BTS) this is acute severe asthma which could be life-threatening. Serial peak flow readings provide information concerning the trend of the patient's large airways and this information can help monitor treatment effects.

SPIROMETRY

The use of spirometry is ever increasing. This is due to several factors, notably the equipment becoming less expensive, smaller and more portable and the increase in the number of respiratory guidelines suggesting that it should be used more widely (BTS 2003). Consequently the use of spirometry in both primary and secondary care is now widespread, but a note of caution needs to be applied: widespread is not always synonymous with the concept that the data obtained is always accurately and correctly interpreted. Rudolf *et al.* (1999) reported that in a survey of primary care-based health professionals 69% of nurses had a spirometer within their practice. However, when presented with a number of traces obtained

Table 8.4 Spirometry respiratory values.

Name of respiratory function measured	Discussion
Vital capacity (VC)	Maximum amount of air that can be exhaled from the lungs after maximal inspiration.
Forced vital capacity (FVC)	The total amount of air that can be forcibly expired from the lungs.
Forced expiratory volume in 1 second (FEV_1)	Amount of air that can be forcibly expired in one second.
Forced expiratory flow (FEF)	Flow of air forced from the lungs. Some spirometers calculate the average flow rate of air during the middle part of the forced expiratory volume $FEF_{25-75\%}$. However this is less reproducible than FEV_1 and makes interpretation difficult.

from spirometry only half of the nurses regularly undertaking this test were able to correctly interpret the spirometry results. The score was lower for GPs, with only a third of them interpreting the results correctly.

Types of spirometer

Flow sensing spirometers are now widely used in clinical care. These spirometers generally utilise a sensor that detects and measures flow by:

- Pressure drop across a resistance (Pneumotach).
- Cooling of a heated wire.
- Electronically counting the rotation of a turbine blade.

These spirometers are widely used in primary care since they are small, calculate respiratory values and may include an interpretation of results (see Fig. 8.5).

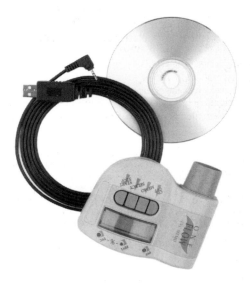

Fig. 8.5 A type of spirometer. Reproduced with permission from Clement Clark.

Performing spirometry tests

The patient must always have the features of the test and the equipment explained to them prior to commencing spirometry testing. This familiarisation phase of the proceedings should include showing them how the equipment works and what it looks like.

Many spirometers have the capacity to calculate a range of respiratory values based upon both predicated values and real values obtained from the patient. In order to achieve this it is usually necessary to input some basic patient related data into the spirometer prior to its use. This usually includes (Pierce & Johns 1995):

- **Patient's age:** up to circa 20 years of age respiratory values generally increase; however over this age all respiratory values usually fall.
- **Height:** the taller the person the greater the respiratory values.
- **Gender:** for a given height and age males will have greater FEV_1, FV and PEFR but a lower FEV_1/ FVC%.
- **Weight.**

In some programs other variables may be considered in the evaluation of the results, e.g.:

- **Ethnic origin.** *FEV_1 and FVC:* Caucasians have the largest volumes; Polynesians have among the lowest volumes; Africans have volumes 10–15% lower than Caucasians of the same age and height since they have a shorter thorax; Chinese have volumes circa 20% lower than similar sized Caucasians; Indians circa 10% lower.

Guidelines for the performance of spirometry have been written (ATS 1987, ATS 1991, ATS 1994) and a summary of these are presented below.

Prior to the test the patient should avoid:

- Vigorous exercise for at least 30 minutes.
- Alcohol for at least 4 hours.
- Wearing tight restrictive clothing.

- Taking of bronchodilators for 6 hours.
- Smoking for 24 hours.
- Patient should be sitting upright or standing, in children the vital capacity is greater when standing.

The test procedure
- Ensure that the spirometer is suitably 'primed' for the test.
- Place a nose peg on patient's nose to occlude nostrils (this is not essential but it is recommended).
- Ask the patient to breathe in fully.
- Seal his/her lips around the mouthpiece.
- Breathe out air as fast and as long as possible.
- Breathe in again as forcibly as possible.

It is essential to ensure:

- That there is a good seal around the mouthpiece.
- That the patient does not lean forward during the test.
- That the expiration and inspiration is undertaken forcibly.

Also, the following should be observed:

1. At least three acceptable results should be obtained, with the highest and second highest FVC agreeing within 0.2 L (Pierce & Johns 1995).
2. Expiration should be at least 6 seconds duration.
3. End of test should indicate no change in volume for at least 1 second after exhalation duration of 6 or more seconds.
4. Spirometer temperature should be between 17 and 40 degrees Celsius.
5. Patient should be sitting or standing.

Spirometers can only measure respiratory volumes that lie within the vital capacity range. In order to measure residual volume, total lung capacity and functional residual volume other techniques are to be employed. These include helium dilution, whole body plethysmography and nitrogen wash-outs. Further information concerning these techniques can be obtained from Bourke (2003).

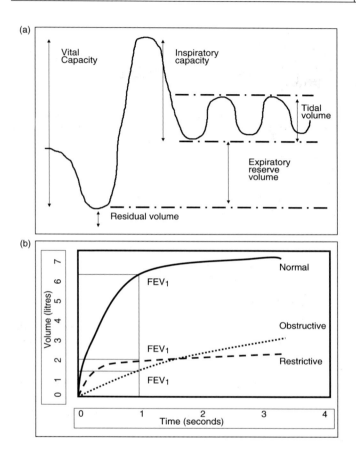

Fig. 8.6a & b Spirometry tracings.

CHEST X-RAYS

Chest X-rays were one of the first medical utilisations of X-ray imaging (Ward *et al.* 2002) and remain today the mainstay of non-invasive diagnostic imaging. Standard two dimensional chest X-rays are used daily to evaluate morphological abnormalities within the chest. Recent advances upon this technique include the development of three dimensional imaging (computed tomography scans) and physiologic images (ventilation perfusion scans).

The most common chest X-ray is a posterior anterior (PA) chest radiograph. Its name indicates the direction in which the X-rays pass through the patient in this case from the back of the patient to the front. It will produce a two-dimensional negative image visualisation of the lungs, great vessels, heart, diaphragm and mediastinum. The patient should be upright and holding their breath while the chest X-ray is taken. In many respiratory illnesses this is impossible to achieve and the skills of the radiographer (in taking the X-ray) and then the radiologist (in analysing the image) are often employed to ensure that the most accurate interpretation of the chest X-ray is obtained.

Figure 8.7 illustrates the major components of an idealised PA chest X-ray.

BREATHLESSNESS SCALES
The experience of breathlessness is variable and depends primarily upon the patient. **Dyspnoea** (is literally translated as *difficulty in breathing* (Ahmedzai 1993). The medical terminology does little to convey what the sensation of 'difficulty in breathing' *means* for the patient, nor the impact that it has upon their daily lives (Andrews 2002). Consequently many 'tools' have been developed that attempt to try and find a method to 'quantify' the experience of breathlessness.

Gift (1990) has designed a visual analogue scale which is comparable to the visual pain scale frequently used in clinical care. Figure 8.8 illustrates Gift's scale; the patient places a mark to indicate their perception of their breathlessness.

However the visual analogue scale is difficult for patients to use and has limited interpretation (Van Der Molen 1995).

Other breathlessness assessment scales are the breathless distress scale and breathless activity scale (Hoyal *et al.* 2002); these should not be used in isolation but in conjunction with nursing assessment documentation (see Tables 8.5 and 8.6).

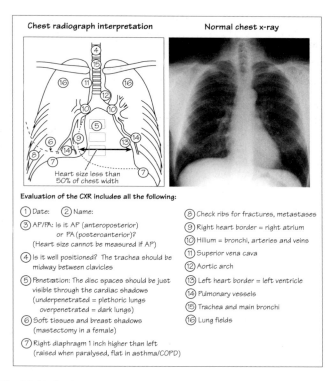

Chest radiograph interpretation

Normal chest x-ray

Heart size less than
50% of chest width

Evaluation of the CXR includes all the following:

1. Date: 2. Name:

3. AP/PA: Is it AP (anteroposterior)
   or PA (posteroanterior)?
   (Heart size cannot be measured if AP)

4. Is it well positioned? The trachea should be
   midway between clavicles

5. Penetration: The disc spaces should be just
   visible through the cardiac shadows
   (underpenetrated = plethoric lungs
   overpenetrated = dark lungs)

6. Soft tissues and breast shadows
   (mastectomy in a female)

7. Right diaphragm 1 inch higher than left
   (raised when paralysed, flat in asthma/COPD)

8. Check ribs for fractures, metastases

9. Right heart border = right atrium

10. Hilum = bronchi, arteries and veins

11. Superior vena cava

12. Aortic arch

13. Left heart border = left ventricle

14. Pulmonary vessels

15. Trachea and main bronchi

16. Lung fields

Fig. 8.7 Idealised chest X-ray. With permission from Blackwell Publishing (Ward 2002).

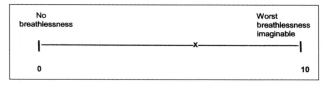

No
breathlessness

Worst
breathlessness
imaginable

X

0   10

Fig. 8.8 Gift pain scale for breathlessness.

Table 8.5 Breathlessness assessment scale (Hoyal *et al.* 2002).

Breathless Distress Scale	Breathless Activity Scale
Please choose the score that best describes the maximum distress you have experienced over the past 24 hours.	*Please choose the score that best describes the maximum level of activity over the past 24 hours.*
0 None at all	0 No breathlessness
1 Some breathlessness, but not troublesome	1 On climbing stairs or hills
2 Breathlessness that is troublesome from time to time	2 On walking more than 100 yards on the flat
3 Breathlessness that is distressing for some of the time	3 On walking less than 100 yards on the flat
4 Breathlessness that is distressing for much of the time	4 On minimum activities, for example dressing, washing
5 Overwhelming breathlessness – can think of nothing else	5 When sitting in a chair or bed
	6 At all times, and feel as if I am fighting for each breath.

Table 8.6 Modified Borg Scale for breathlessness assessment. (Kendrick *et al.* 2000).

0	No breathlessness at all
0.5	Very, very slight (just noticeable)
1	Very slight
2	Slight breathlessness
3	Modified
4	Somewhat severe
5	Severe breathlessness
6	
7	Very severe breathlessness
8	
9	Very, very severe (almost maximal)
10	Maximal

(Kendrick *et al.* 2000).

Another scale (The Borg scale) and the modified version shown in Table 8.6, has been found to be useful in acute clinical situations, such as accident and emergency department. It is quick and easy for clinical staff to use and provides rapid information concerning the patient assessment and clinical decision making.

MEASUREMENT OF FUNCTIONAL HEALTH STATUS OF PATIENTS IN RESPIRATORY CONDITIONS

The measurement of symptoms, and their impact upon quality of life and functional ability of the patients can be measured using a number of functional health questionnaires. These include: *St George's respiratory questionnaire* (SGRQ) developed by Professor Jones; *Asthma quality of life questionnaire* (developed by Juniper *et al.*); Guyatt's McMaster *Chronic respiratory questionnaire* (CRQ).

In essence the choice of functional health status questionnaire will depend upon the preliminary or confirmed diagnosis, the most suitable for a specific patient and the adopted policy of the clinic.

All these questionnaires require a high degree of literacy and patient compliance; some of them can be self-administered and thus remove the necessity for a clinician's presence. They should be used more frequently in clinical practice since the information revealed can provide a means of monitoring patient's condition and its response to treatment.

DOCUMENTATION

Patient assessment is carried out continuously in all interactions between clinicians and patients. All patient-related information should be appropriately documented and recorded contemporaneously. Information related to respiratory functioning can be gathered together from a myriad of sources, patient and family, health professionals and from your own clinical observation. Many respiratory conditions will necessitate the patient having repeated contact with health professionals and frequent monitoring of their condition. This practice can only be effected efficiently and speedily by the opportunity to review clear, detailed, organised documentation of previous respiratory assessments.

Documentation is central to maintaining patient effective communication and continuity of patient care. Documentation should include what has been discerned from the patient's physical assessment and any deviations from the normal should always be documented. All interventions should be clearly recorded, whether nursing, medical, or any physiotherapy provided and include all the information given to patient and family. Evaluation of previous interventions should also appear in the notes.

Poor or incomplete documentation can be detrimental to good patient care. It is possible that patients can receive or feel they have received inadequate patient care, despite repeated interventions and treatment. They may have missed clinical appointments for treatment and interventions and have deteriorated in their respiratory condition. Without documentation, comparison to their previous respiratory condition is not possible. Arguably the situation in a court of law is that if events are not documented and recorded suitably, then no proof exists that they occurred. Ensure that all documentation is complete and filled in appropriately: this is a crucial part of the care of all patients.

SUMMARY

This chapter has outlined the following principles:

❏ Respiratory patient assessment including observation of the patient and patient examination.
❏ Use and abuses of pulse oximetry.
❏ Arterial blood gas analysis.
❏ Measurement of peak expiratory flow rate.
❏ Use of spirometry and common traces obtained.
❏ Basic interpretation of a normal chest X-ray.
❏ Breathlessness scales and respiratory health assessment.
❏ Importance of documentation.

REFERENCES

Ahern J, Philpot P (2002) Assessing acutely ill patients on general wards. *Nursing Standard* **16** (47): 54–57.

Ahmedzi S (1993) Palliation of respiratory symptoms. In: Doyle D *et al.* (eds) *Oxford textbook of palliative medicine*. Oxford University Press, Oxford.

American Thoracic Society (1987) Standardization of spirometry. *American Review of Respiratory Disease* **136**: 1285–1295.

American Thoracic Society (1991) Lung function testing: selection of references values and interpretive strategies. *American Review of Respiratory Disease* **144**: 1202–1218.

American Thoracic Society (1994) Standardization of spirometry. *American Journal of Respiratory and Critical Care Medicine* **152**: 1107–1136.

Andrews T (2002) The management of breathlessness in palliative care. *Nursing Standard* **17** (5): 43–52.

Barkauskas V, Stolenberg-Allen K, Baumann L, Darling-Fisher C (1994) *Health and physical assessment*. Mosby, London.

Bennett C (2002) Respiratory care. In: Workman B, Bennett C. *Key nursing skills*. Whurr, London.

Bourke SJ (2003) *Respiratory medicine*. Blackwell Publishing, Oxford.

British Thoracic Society, Scottish Intercollegiate Guidelines Network, National Asthma Campaign, British Association for Accident and Emergency Medicine, General Practice in Airways Group, Royal College of Paediatrics and Child Health, Royal College of Physicians of London (2003) British Guideline on the Management of Asthma. A national clinical guideline. *Thorax* **58** (Suppl. 1):i1–i94.

Carter BG, Carlin JB, Tibballs J *et al.* (1998) Accuracy of two pulse oximeters at low arterial hemoglobin-oxygen saturation. *Critical Care Medicine* **26** (6): 1128–1133.

Clutton-Brock T (1997) The assessment and monitoring of respiratory function. In: Goldhill D, Withington P (eds) *Textbook of intensive care*. Chapman & Hall, London.

Cox CL (1997) *Advanced practice: physical assessment*. City University, London.

Darovic GO, (1997) Physical assessment of the pulmonary system. In: Darovic GO (ed.) *Hemodynamic monitoring: invasive and noninvasive clinical application*, 2nd edn. Philadelphia, WB Saunders.

Dobson F (1993) Shedding light on pulse oximetry. *Nursing Standard* **7** (46): 4–11.

Gift A (1990) Dyspnea. *Nursing Clinics of North America* **25** (4): 955–956.

Goldhill DR, White SA, Sumner A (1999) Physiological values and procedures in the 24 hours before ICU admission from the ward. *Anaesthesia* **54** (6): 529–534.

Guyatt GH, Berman LB, Townsend M *et al.* (1987) A measure of quality of life for clinical trials in chronic lung disease. *Thorax* **42**: 773–778.

Harrahill M (1991) Pulse oximetry, pearls and pitfalls. *Journal of Emergency Nursing* **17** (6): 437–439.

Hinds CJ, Watson D (1996) *Intensive care: a concise textbook*, 2nd edn. WB Saunders, London.

Hope R *et al.* (1998) *Oxford handbook of clinical medicine*, 4th edn. Oxford University Press, Oxford.

Jevon P, Ewens B (2001) Assessment of a breathless patient. *Nursing Standard* **15** (16): 48–53.

Jones PW (1991) Quality of life measurement for patients with diseases of the airways. *Thorax* **46**: 676–682.

Junniper EF *et al.* (1992) Evaluation of impairment of health related quality of life in asthma: development of a questionnaire for use in clinical trials. *Thorax* **47**: 76–83.

Kendrick AH, Smith EC (1992) Respiratory measurements 2: interpreting simple measurements of lung function. *Professional Nurse* **7** (11): 748–754.

Kendrick K, Baxi S, Smith R (2000) Usefulness of the modified 0–10 Borg scale in assessing the degree of dyspnoea in patients with COPD and asthma. *Journal of Emergency Nursing* **26** (3): 216–222.

Pierce R, Johns DP (1995) *Spirometry handbook.* National Asthma Council, Melbourne, Australia.

Pitkin AD, Roberts CM, Wedzicha JA (1994) Arterialised earlobe blood gas analysis: an underused technique. *Thorax* **49**: 364–366.

Ralston AC *et al.* (1992) Potential errors in pulse oximetry. *Anaesthesia* **46** (4): 291–295.

Ruch V (1999) pulmonary disorders. In: Gawlinski A, Hamwi D (eds) *Acute care nurse practitioner, clinical curriculum and certification review.* WB Saunders, Philadelphia.

Rudolf M, Buchanan A, Hart L (1999) Making spirometry happen. *Thorax* **54** (Suppl. 5): S1–S28.

Seidal H, Ball J, Danins J, Benedict G (1995) *Mosby's guide to physical examination*, 3rd edn. Mosby, London.

Sheehy S, Lombardi J (1995) *Emergency care*, 4th edn. Mosby, St Louis, Mo.

Stoneham MD, *et al.* (1994) Knowledge about pulse oximetry among medical and nursing staff. *Lancet* **344** (8933): 1339–1342.

Wahr J, Tremper K (1996) Oxygen measurement and monitoring techniques. In: Prys-Roberts C, Brown B Jr (eds) *International practice of anaesthesia.* Butterworth, Heinemann, Oxford.

Ward JPT, Ward J, Wiener CM, Leach RM (2002) *The respiratory system at a glance.* Blackwell Science, Oxford.

Woodrow P (1999) Pulse oximetry. *Nursing Standard* **7** (13): 42–46.

Woodrow P (2002) Assessing respiratory function in older people. *Nursing Older People* **14** (3): 27–28.

Appendix A
Spirometry Respiratory Values

Normal predicted spirometry for Caucasian males and females (reproduced with permission from Vitalograph Ltd)

E.R.S. 1993

FEMALE PREDICTED NORMAL VALUES

Age	Height (cm)	150	155	160	165	170	175	180	185	190	195
18 -	FVC	3.11	3.33	3.55	3.77	3.99	4.21	4.43	4.66	4.88	5.10
25	FEV1	2.70	2.90	3.10	3.29	3.49	3.69	3.89	4.08	4.28	4.48
25	FEV1%	84%	84%	84%	84%	84%	84%	84%	84%	84%	84%
25	FEF 25-75%	3.95	4.01	4.07	4.13	4.20	4.26	4.32	4.38	4.45	4.51
25	PEF	383	400	416	433	449	466	482	499	515	532
26 -	FVC	3.00	3.22	3.44	3.67	3.89	4.11	4.33	4.55	4.77	4.99
29	FEV1	2.60	2.80	3.00	3.19	3.39	3.59	3.79	3.98	4.18	4.38
29	FEV1%	84%	84%	84%	84%	84%	84%	84%	84%	84%	84%
29	FEF 25-75%	3.81	3.87	3.93	4.00	4.06	4.12	4.18	4.25	4.31	4.37
29	PEF	376	393	409	426	442	459	475	492	508	525
29 -	FVC	2.90	3.12	3.34	3.56	3.78	4.00	4.23	4.45	4.67	4.89
33	FEV1	2.50	2.70	2.90	3.09	3.29	3.49	3.69	3.88	4.08	4.28
33	FEV1%	83%	83%	83%	83%	83%	83%	83%	83%	83%	83%
33	FEF 25-75%	3.67	3.74	3.80	3.86	3.92	3.99	4.05	4.11	4.17	4.24
33	PEF	369	386	402	419	435	452	468	485	501	518

Age	Height (cm)	150	155	160	165	170	175	180	185	190	195
34 -	FVC	2.79	3.01	3.24	3.46	3.68	3.90	4.12	4.34	4.57	4.79
37	FEV1	2.40	2.60	2.80	2.99	3.19	3.39	3.59	3.78	3.98	4.18
37	FEV1%	82%	82%	82%	82%	82%	82%	82%	82%	82%	82%
37	FEF 25-75%	3.54	3.60	3.66	3.72	3.79	3.85	3.91	3.97	4.04	4.10
37	PEF	362	378	395	411	428	444	461	477	494	510
38 -	FVC	2.69	2.91	3.13	3.35	3.58	3.80	4.02	4.24	4.46	4.68
41	FEV1	2.30	2.50	2.70	2.89	3.09	3.29	3.49	3.68	3.88	4.08
41	FEV1%	81%	81%	81%	81%	81%	81%	81%	81%	81%	81%
41	FEF 25-75%	3.40	3.46	3.53	3.59	3.65	3.71	3.78	3.84	3.90	3.96
41	PEF	355	371	388	404	421	437	454	470	487	503
42 -	FVC	2.59	2.81	3.03	3.25	3.47	3.69	3.91	4.14	4.36	4.58
45	FEV1	2.20	2.40	2.60	2.79	2.99	3.19	3.39	3.58	3.78	3.98
45	FEV1%	81%	81%	81%	81%	81%	81%	81%	81%	81%	81%
45	FEF 25-75%	3.27	3.33	3.39	3.45	3.52	3.58	3.64	3.70	3.77	3.83
45	PEF	347	364	380	397	413	430	446	463	479	496
46 -	FVC	2.48	2.70	2.92	3.15	3.37	3.59	3.81	4.03	4.25	4.47
49	FEV1	2.10	2.30	2.50	2.69	2.89	3.09	3.29	3.48	3.68	3.88
49	FEV1%	80%	80%	80%	80%	80%	80%	80%	80%	80%	80%
49	FEF 25-75%	3.13	3.19	3.25	3.32	3.38	3.44	3.50	3.57	3.63	3.69
49	PEF	340	357	373	390	406	423	439	456	472	489

Age	Height (cm)	150	155	160	165	170	175	180	185	190	195
50 -											
53	FVC	2.38	2.60	2.82	3.04	3.26	3.48	3.71	3.93	4.15	4.37
53	FEV1	2.00	2.20	2.40	2.59	2.79	2.99	3.19	3.38	3.58	3.78
53	FEV1%	79%	79%	79%	79%	79%	79%	79%	79%	79%	79%
53	FEF 25-75%	2.99	3.06	3.12	3.18	3.24	3.31	3.37	3.43	3.49	3.56
53	PEF	333	350	366	383	399	416	432	449	465	482
54 -											
57	FVC	2.27	2.49	2.72	2.94	3.16	3.38	3.60	3.82	4.05	4.27
57	FEV1	1.90	2.10	2.30	2.49	2.69	2.89	3.09	3.28	3.48	3.68
57	FEV1%	78%	78%	78%	78%	78%	78%	78%	78%	78%	78%
57	FEF 25-75%	2.86	2.92	2.98	3.04	3.11	3.17	3.23	3.29	3.36	3.42
57	PEF	326	342	359	375	392	408	425	441	458	474
58 -											
61	FVC	2.17	2.39	2.61	2.83	3.06	3.28	3.50	3.72	3.94	4.16
61	FEV1	1.80	2.00	2.20	2.39	2.59	2.79	2.99	3.18	3.38	3.58
61	FEV1%	78%	78%	78%	78%	78%	78%	78%	78%	78%	78%
61	FEF 25-75%	2.72	2.78	2.85	2.91	2.97	3.03	3.10	3.16	3.22	3.28
61	PEF	319	335	352	368	385	401	418	434	451	467
62 -											
65	FVC	2.07	2.29	2.51	2.73	2.95	3.17	3.39	3.62	3.84	4.06
65	FEV1	1.70	1.90	2.10	2.29	2.49	2.69	2.89	3.08	3.28	3.48
65	FEV1%	77%	77%	77%	77%	77%	77%	77%	77%	77%	77%
65	FEF 25-75%	2.59	2.65	2.71	2.77	2.84	2.90	2.96	3.02	3.09	3.15
65	PEF	311	328	344	361	377	394	410	427	443	460
66 -											
69	FVC	1.96	2.18	2.40	2.63	2.85	3.07	3.29	3.51	3.73	3.95
69	FEV1	1.60	1.80	2.00	2.19	2.39	2.59	2.79	2.98	3.18	3.38
69	FEV1%	76%	76%	76%	76%	76%	76%	76%	76%	76%	76%
69	FEF 25-75%	2.45	2.51	2.57	2.64	2.70	2.76	2.82	2.89	2.95	3.01
69	PEF	304	321	337	354	370	387	403	420	436	453

E.R.S. 1993

MALE PREDICTED NORMAL VALUES

	Age	Height (cm)	150	155	160	165	170	175	180	185	190	195
18 -	25	FVC	3.65	3.94	4.23	4.51	4.80	5.09	5.38	5.67	5.95	6.24
	25	FEV1	3.24	3.45	3.67	3.88	4.10	4.31	4.53	4.74	4.96	5.17
	25	FEV1%	83%	83%	83%	83%	83%	83%	83%	83%	83%	83%
	25	FEF 25-75%	4.54	4.63	4.73	4.83	4.92	5.02	5.12	5.21	5.31	5.41
	25	PEF	497	516	534	552	571	589	608	626	644	663
26 -	29	FVC	3.55	3.83	4.12	4.41	4.70	4.99	5.27	5.56	5.85	6.14
	29	FEV1	3.12	3.33	3.55	3.76	3.98	4.19	4.41	4.62	4.84	5.05
	29	FEV1%	82%	82%	82%	82%	82%	82%	82%	82%	82%	82%
	29	FEF 25-75%	4.36	4.46	4.56	4.65	4.75	4.85	4.95	5.04	5.14	5.24
	29	PEF	487	505	524	542	560	579	597	616	634	653
29 -	33	FVC	3.44	3.73	4.02	4.31	4.59	4.88	5.17	5.46	5.75	6.03
	33	FEV1	3.00	3.22	3.43	3.65	3.86	4.08	4.29	4.51	4.72	4.94
	33	FEV1%	81%	81%	81%	81%	81%	81%	81%	81%	81%	81%
	33	FEF 25-75%	4.19	4.29	4.39	4.48	4.58	4.68	4.77	4.87	4.97	5.06
	33	PEF	476	495	513	532	550	569	587	605	624	642

Age	Height (cm)	150	155	160	165	170	175	180	185	190	195
37	FVC	3.34	3.63	3.91	4.20	4.49	4.78	5.07	5.35	5.64	5.93
37	FEV1	2.89	3.10	3.32	3.53	3.75	3.96	4.18	4.39	4.61	4.82
37	FEV1%	81%	81%	81%	81%	81%	81%	81%	81%	81%	81%
37	FEF 25-75%	4.02	4.12	4.21	4.31	4.41	4.50	4.60	4.70	4.80	4.89
37	PEF	466	485	503	521	540	558	577	595	614	632
41	FVC	3.23	3.52	3.81	4.10	4.39	4.67	4.96	5.25	5.54	5.83
41	FEV1	2.77	2.99	3.20	3.42	3.63	3.85	4.06	4.28	4.49	4.71
41	FEV1%	80%	80%	80%	80%	80%	80%	80%	80%	80%	80%
41	FEF 25-75%	3.85	3.94	4.04	4.14	4.24	4.33	4.43	4.53	4.62	4.72
41	PEF	456	474	493	511	530	548	566	585	603	622
45	FVC	3.13	3.42	3.71	3.99	4.28	4.57	4.86	5.15	5.43	5.72
45	FEV1	2.66	2.87	3.09	3.30	3.52	3.73	3.95	4.16	4.38	4.59
45	FEV1%	79%	79%	79%	79%	79%	79%	79%	79%	79%	79%
45	FEF 25-75%	3.68	3.77	3.87	3.97	4.06	4.16	4.26	4.35	4.45	4.55
45	PEF	446	464	482	501	519	538	556	574	593	611
49	FVC	3.03	3.31	3.60	3.89	4.18	4.47	4.75	5.04	5.33	5.62
49	FEV1	2.54	2.75	2.97	3.18	3.40	3.61	3.83	4.04	4.26	4.47
49	FEV1%	78%	78%	78%	78%	78%	78%	78%	78%	78%	78%
49	FEF 25-75%	3.50	3.60	3.70	3.79	3.89	3.99	4.09	4.18	4.28	4.38
49	PEF	435	454	472	490	509	527	546	564	583	601
53	FVC	2.92	3.21	3.50	3.79	4.07	4.36	4.65	4.94	5.23	5.51
53	FEV1	2.42	2.64	2.85	3.07	3.28	3.50	3.71	3.93	4.14	4.36
53	FEV1%	78%	78%	78%	78%	78%	78%	78%	78%	78%	78%
53	FEF 25-75%	3.33	3.43	3.53	3.62	3.72	3.82	3.91	4.01	4.11	4.20
53	PEF	425	443	462	480	499	517	535	554	572	591

Age brackets (left margin): 34 -, 38 -, 42 -, 46 -, 50 -

Age	Height (cm)	150	155	160	165	170	175	180	185	190	195
54 -											
57	FVC	2.82	3.11	3.39	3.68	3.97	4.26	4.55	4.83	5.12	5.41
57	FEV1	2.31	2.52	2.74	2.95	3.17	3.38	3.60	3.81	4.03	4.24
57	FEV1%	77%	77%	77%	77%	77%	77%	77%	77%	77%	77%
57	FEF 25-75%	3.16	3.26	3.35	3.45	3.55	3.64	3.74	3.84	3.94	4.03
57	PEF	415	433	451	470	488	507	525	543	562	580
58 -											
61	FVC	2.71	3.00	3.29	3.58	3.87	4.15	4.44	4.73	5.02	5.31
61	FEV1	2.19	2.41	2.62	2.84	3.05	3.27	3.48	3.70	3.91	4.13
61	FEV1%	76%	76%	76%	76%	76%	76%	76%	76%	76%	76%
61	FEF 25-75%	2.99	3.08	3.18	3.28	3.38	3.47	3.57	3.67	3.76	3.86
61	PEF	404	423	441	459	478	496	515	533	552	570
62 -											
65	FVC	2.61	2.90	3.19	3.47	3.76	4.05	4.34	4.63	4.91	5.20
65	FEV1	2.08	2.29	2.51	2.72	2.94	3.15	3.37	3.58	3.80	4.01
65	FEV1%	76%	76%	76%	76%	76%	76%	76%	76%	76%	76%
65	FEF 25-75%	2.82	2.91	3.01	3.11	3.20	3.30	3.40	3.49	3.59	3.69
65	PEF	394	412	431	449	468	486	504	523	541	560
66 -											
69	FVC	2.51	2.79	3.08	3.37	3.66	3.95	4.23	4.52	4.81	5.10
69	FEV1	1.96	2.17	2.39	2.60	2.82	3.03	3.25	3.46	3.68	3.89
69	FEV1%	75%	75%	75%	75%	75%	75%	75%	75%	75%	75%
69	FEF 25-75%	2.64	2.74	2.84	2.93	3.03	3.13	3.23	3.32	3.42	3.52
69	PEF	384	402	420	439	457	476	494	513	531	549

PREDICTED NORMAL VALUES – CHILDREN

Male

Height (cm)	100	102	104	106	108	110	112	114	116	118
FVC	0.96	1.01	1.07	1.12	1.18	1.24	1.30	1.37	1.43	1.50
FEV1	0.84	0.88	0.93	0.98	1.04	1.09	1.15	1.21	1.27	1.33
FEV1%	87%	87%	87%	88%	88%	88%	88%	88%	89%	89%
FEF 25-75%	0.91	0.99	1.08	1.17	1.26	1.34	1.43	1.52	1.61	1.69
PEF	100	110	121	131	142	152	163	173	184	194

Height (cm)	120	122	124	126	128	130	132	134	136	138
FVC	1.57	1.64	1.71	1.78	1.86	1.94	2.02	2.10	2.19	2.27
FEV1	1.39	1.46	1.53	1.60	1.67	1.74	1.82	1.90	1.98	2.06
FEV1%	89%	89%	89%	89%	90%	90%	90%	90%	90%	91%
FEF 25-75%	1.78	1.87	1.95	2.04	2.13	2.22	2.30	2.39	2.48	2.57
PEF	205	215	226	236	247	257	268	278	289	299

Height (cm)	140	142	144	146	148	150	152	154	156	158
FVC	2.36	2.46	2.55	2.64	2.74	2.84	2.94	3.05	3.16	3.26
FEV1	2.14	2.23	2.32	2.41	2.51	2.60	2.70	2.80	2.90	3.01
FEV1%	91%	91%	91%	91%	91%	92%	92%	92%	92%	92%
FEF 25-75%	2.65	2.74	2.83	2.92	3.00	3.09	3.18	3.27	3.35	3.44
PEF	310	320	331	341	352	362	373	383	394	404

Height (cm)	160	162	164	166	168	170	172	174	176	178
FVC	3.38	3.49	3.61	3.73	3.85	3.97	4.10	4.22	4.35	4.49
FEV1	3.12	3.23	3.34	3.46	3.57	3.69	3.82	3.94	4.07	4.20
FEV1%	92%	92%	93%	93%	93%	93%	93%	93%	93%	94%
FEF 25-75%	3.53	3.61	3.70	3.79	3.88	3.96	4.05	4.14	4.23	4.31
PEF	415	425	436	446	456	467	477	488	498	509

Height (cm)	180	182	184	186	188	190	192	194	196	198
FVC	4.62	4.76	4.90	5.05	5.19	5.34	5.49	5.65	5.80	5.96
FEV1	4.33	4.47	4.61	4.75	4.90	5.04	5.19	5.35	5.50	5.66
FEV1%	94%	94%	93%	94%	94%	94%	95%	95%	95%	95%
FEF 25-75%	4.40	4.49	4.58	4.66	4.75	4.84	4.92	5.01	5.10	5.19
PEF	519	530	540	551	561	572	582	593	603	614

Female

Height (cm)	100	102	104	106	108	110	112	114	116	118
FVC	0.91	0.96	1.01	1.06	1.12	1.18	1.24	1.30	1.36	1.43
FEV1	0.84	0.88	0.93	0.98	1.04	1.09	1.15	1.21	1.27	1.33
FEV1%	92%	92%	92%	92%	93%	93%	93%	93%	93%	93%
FEF 25-75%	0.91	0.99	1.08	1.17	1.26	1.34	1.43	1.52	1.61	1.69
PEF	100	110	121	131	142	152	163	173	184	194

Height (cm)	120	122	124	126	128	130	132	134	136	138
FVC	1.49	1.56	1.63	1.70	1.78	1.86	1.93	2.01	2.10	2.18
FEV1	1.39	1.46	1.53	1.60	1.67	1.74	1.82	1.90	1.98	2.06
FEV1%	93%	93%	94%	94%	94%	94%	94%	94%	94%	94%
FEF 25-75%	1.78	1.87	1.95	2.04	2.13	2.22	2.30	2.39	2.48	2.57
PEF	205	215	226	236	247	257	268	278	289	299

Height (cm)	140	142	144	146	148	150	152	154	156	158
FVC	2.27	2.36	2.45	2.54	2.64	2.74	2.84	2.94	3.05	3.15
FEV1	2.14	2.23	2.32	2.41	2.51	2.60	2.70	2.80	2.90	3.01
FEV1%	94%	95%	95%	95%	95%	95%	95%	95%	95%	95%
FEF 25-75%	2.65	2.74	2.83	2.92	3.00	3.09	3.18	3.27	3.35	3.44
PEF	310	320	331	341	352	362	373	383	394	404

Height (cm)	160	162	164	166	168	170	172	174	176	178
FVC	3.26	3.38	3.49	3.61	3.73	3.85	3.97	4.10	4.23	4.36
FEV1	3.12	3.23	3.34	3.46	3.57	3.69	3.82	3.94	4.07	4.20
FEV1%	96%	96%	96%	96%	96%	96%	96%	96%	96%	96%
FEF 25-75%	3.53	3.61	3.70	3.79	3.88	3.96	4.05	4.14	4.23	4.31
PEF	415	425	436	446	456	467	477	488	498	509

Height (cm)	180	182	184	186	188	190	192	194	196	198
FVC	4.50	4.63	4.77	4.92	5.06	5.21	5.36	5.51	5.67	5.83
FEV1	4.33	4.47	4.61	4.75	4.90	5.04	5.19	5.35	5.50	5.66
FEV1%	96%	96%	97%	97%	97%	97%	97%	97%	97%	97%
FEF 25-75%	4.40	4.49	4.58	4.66	4.75	4.84	4.92	5.01	5.10	5.19
PEF	519	530	540	551	561	572	582	593	603	614

Appendix B
Pharmaceutical Companies and Respiratory Product Manufacturers

Name	Address/ contact details
Air Products Plc	Weston Road
	Crewe Cheshire CW1 6BT
	0800 373 580
Astrazeneca	www.astrazeneca.com
BOC	www.boc.com
Boehringer Ingelheim	www.boehringer-ingelheim.com
Clement Clarke International Ltd.	Edinburgh Way
	Harlow Essex
	CM20 2TT
	01279 414969
	www.clement-clarke.com
Farraris	www.farrarismedical.com
GlaxoSmithKline	GlaxoWellcome UK Ltd.
	Stockley Park West
	Uxbridge Middlesex UB11 1BT
	Customerservices@glaxowellcome.co.uk
	0800 22 1441
Merck Sharp & Dohme Ltd	Hertford Road
	Hoddesdon Hertfordshire EN11 9BU
Vitalograph	www.vitalograph.co.uk

Appendix C
Smoking Cessation Advice

Name	Contact details	Information provided
ASH (Action on Smoking and Health)	020 7739 5902 www.ash.org.uk	For both health professionals and the public.
QUIT	0800 002 200 www.stopsmoking@quit.org.uk www.quit.org.uk	Smoking cessation advice for the public.
NHS smoking cessation website	www.doh.nhsweb.nhs.uk/ nhssmokingcessation/	For both the public and health professionals.

Appendix D
Respiratory Charities

Name	Address	Range of products/ resources available
British Lung Foundation	78 Hatton Garden London EC1N 8JR 020 7831 5831 info@britishlungfoundation.com www.lunguk.org	Patient-centred leaflets and information sheets. Information for health professionals. Research funding.
Asthma UK (formally National Asthma Campaign)	www.asthma.org.uk	Patient-centred leaflets, health professional information and research funding.
National Asthma Campaign Scotland	2a North Charlotte Street Edinburgh EH2 4HR	As above.
Action Asthma patient service	www.actionasthma.co.uk provided by Allen & Hanburys respiratory division of GSK.	Patient help lines and leaflets.
Allergy UK	www.allergyuk.org	Will produce translation cards for patients to carry in case of emergency treatment when abroad.

Appendix E
Professional Societies/Education and Training Organisations

Name	Contact details
British Thoracic Society	www.brit-thoracic.org.uk
American Thoracic Society	www.thoracic.org
Respiratory Education and Training Centres	www.respiratoryetc.com
Association of Respiratory Nurse Specialists	www.arns.co.uk
Royal College of Nurses – Respiratory Forum	www.rcn.org.uk
European Respiratory Society	www.ersnet.org
General Practice Airways Group	www.gpiag-asthma.org/GPIAG
National Respiratory Training Centre	www.nrtc.org.uk
Global Initiative for Asthma (GINA)	www.ginasthma.com
Lung and Asthma Information Agency	www.sghma.ac.uk/depts/phs/laia/laia.htm

Index